PRAISE FOR THE BOOK...

Dr. Panwalker understands, deeply, the pain and suffering of patients and healthcare workers alike. Many decades of experience taking care of patients in our broken healthcare system have given him tremendous insight into the causes and solutions to our problems. *Sick and Scared* provides a path forward, step by step, for our patients, healthcare workers, and policymakers to fix US healthcare. A must read!

~ Brad Spellberg MD, FACP, Chief Medical officer, Los Angeles County and University of Southern California Medical Center; Author of "Broken, Bankrupt and Dying."

Anand Panwalker lays bare the myths, sacred cows, and foibles of modern medicine while celebrating its joys, aspirational intent, and even its challenges. This book is informative and well-informed; poetic in places yet crystalline in its clarity. We must do better, the author exhorts, and rightly so. This is a must-read for anyone involved in or affected by medical care in the US.

~ Omar Khan MD, President & CEO, Delaware Health Sciences Alliance; Editor-in-Chief, Delaware Journal of Public Health; Faculty, University of Pennsylvania and Sidney Kimmel College of Medicine and the Co-Author of "Readings in Global Health;" "The End of Polio" and "Megacities & Global Health."

A tour de force of scholarship. Loved the book. Articulates masterfully the feelings we share. But it is more than that. The author writes beautifully. The tips are useful reminders. The litany of catastrophes is harrowing but very useful. Both doctors and lay persons will benefit from reading this book.

~ Bennett Lorber MD. D.Sc. Emeritus Professor, Temple University School of Medicine, Philadelphia.

Incredibly powerful exposition of all the problems we have with expensive and fragmented healthcare in the wealthiest county in the world; heartfelt writing from someone who has practiced Medicine on three continents.

~ Dean Winslow MD. Professor of Medicine, Stanford University. Colonel, U.S. Air Force (retired)

Over two generations, we have seen medical care become increasingly effective at addressing specific diseases. Discontent on the part of patients and their doctors has expanded amid this technical glory. Dr. Panwalker draws on a professional lifetime of effort and experience to masterfully explain the sources of apprehension of patients and frustration of doctors that has emerged and impart his immense insight on potential remedies

~ Richard Plotzker MD. Endocrinologist, Newark, Delaware.

The author is the senior leader for professional excellence at one of the country's top healthcare systems. He is the "doctor's doctor" to whom family, friends and fellow doctors turn for his valued judgment and counsel. Now everyone can benefit from his guidance and wisdom by reading this eye-opening book!

~ Vijay Sathe MBA, PhD. The C. S. & D. J. Davidson Chair and Professor of Management at the Drucker School, Claremont, California.

A brutally honest critique of our healthcare system which has resulted in the erosion of the physician-patient relationship, physician burnout, and increasing financial stress for families. Fortunately, Dr. Panwalker's book not only covers the flaws of our system but also provides us with a variety of potential solutions. This is truly a good read!

~ James Malow MD, Former Chairman, Department of Medicine, Illinois Masonic Hospital, and Professor at Rush Medical School, Chicago.

This wonderful book is an almost-impossible empathetic critique of today's healthcare system. Admirably fair-minded with the aim to inspire all involved to be their best human selves...by being mindful of one another. A great service for every sector of the health care industry.

The great hallmark- empathy! - shines through every concern, criticism, and suggestion for improvement! The only possible response for this Herculean achievement is joyful gratitude!

~ Chuck Selvaggio, Executive Director, Neighbors to Nicaragua, Inc., Delaware.

Anand Panwalker has artfully and thoughtfully created an honest, introspective review of the current state of our woefully inadequate US medical system-and then created a blueprint for how both patients and clinicians can work together to improve it for the future. His voice is quietly but pointedly "calling us out" that we can and must do better than this.

~ David Bercaw MD, FAAFP. Department of Family Medicine, Christiana Care.

The American health system is broken. Most of us know that, but only some offer solutions. Anand Panwalker provides a unique perspective: a brilliant infectious disease physician who has practiced on three continents and has made the United States his home for many decades. His blunt diagnoses of our American health system may sting, but the author provides all of us a way forward that incorporates caring, compassion and good medicine

~ Christopher Haines MD, Assistant Professor, Department of Family and Community Medicine and Department of Medical Physiology and Biophysics, Sidney Kimmel College of Medicine, Philadelphia.

Sick and Scared has taken on the daunting task of describing the shortcomings and failures of the American healthcare system and has done so with unwavering candor. It is a well-researched and thoroughly referenced book. A "must read" not only for medical professionals but also for lay people.

~ Vijay Abhyankar MD, Internist and Assistant Vice-president for Medical affairs at the University of Maryland Upper Chesapeake Medical Center, Bel Air, Maryland.

An excellent, cogent review of the current status of healthcare, including the frustrations for patients and physicians. Should be required reading for all medical students and residents. Many valuable tips for patients and physicians.

~ G. Wesley White MD., Infectious Disease Physician, Chicago.

The book is packed with real-life anecdotes and ends with practical tips for patients, physicians, administrators and ideas for health care reform. I highly recommend this highly readable opus to anyone who is interested in improving their own health and the health care system in USA

~ Avinash Chitnis B.Sc.- Scientist, Engineer, Corporate Manager-Telecommunications (Retired)

Very timely. In times of heightened tensions & political dysfunction, the book comes across as concerned, considerate, and full of empathy for care seekers & care givers. This book should be very helpful for people contemplating a career in the medical profession. A compelling narrative.

~ Kumar Fanse MS, Senior Manager, Bechtel Corporation (Retired); Community Leader and Volunteer, Alameda, California.

It is not his first book. His highly successful memoir, *A Place of Cold Water*, draws attention to the history of discrimination faced by graduates of non-U.S. medical schools regardless of their actual ability. Sick and Scared casts a wider net, encompassing not only that issue, but also such themes as over-reliance on a flawed system of electronic medical records, administrative bloat, and medical errors. It is meticulously researched, with almost 300 citations. It draws on the author's own experience as a physician, patient, and family caregiver, as well as on communications from colleagues. Although the message is a troubling one, it cannot be ignored

~ Joan DelFattore, BA, MA, MS, PhD. Professor Emerita, English and Legal studies University of Delaware. Author of three books with Yale University.

The purpose of this book is to diagnose and treat the malady within health care. The author empathizes with caregivers/care seekers and suggests practical approaches for reform. A sincere, lucid and organized documentation of wisdom earned through fifty years of professional experience.

~ Sitara Jabeen, M.A., English literature, Author, Journalist (Dhaka Tribune) and College professor.

Dr. Panwalker's knowledge, experience, compassion, and love for his profession are unequivocal as he proposes tips for patients and physicians as well as possible solutions to reform our dysfunctional health-care system. A brilliant doctor's effort to bring back, "noble," to his profession.

~ Shefali Kapoor Dhir B.A. (Economics) BA (Business Administration). Montessori Teacher, Ursuline Academy, Wilmington, Delaware.

A must read, self-help book for the "sick and the scared and the confused" just in time during this pandemic. Painstakingly and meticulously researched; very comprehensive and written by an expert with a heart.

~ Vijaya Balchandani B.Ed, B.Sc, M.Sc, Teacher

Doctor Panwalker has painted a stark portrait of the current dysfunctional state of health care based on his personal experiences as a clinician as well as an administrator. This well researched book offers survival tips for both patients and physicians

~ Bala Carver MD. State College, Pennsylvania.

SICK
AND
SCARED

AN ESSENTIAL GUIDE FOR PATIENTS AND DOCTORS

100 tips for patient safety
66 tips for physician wellness
Seven steps to healthcare reform

ANAND PANWALKER, M.D.

Copyright © 2020 by Anand Panwalker, M.D.

All rights reserved. This book or any portion thereof may not be reproduced or used in any manner whatsoever without the express written permission of the author except for the use of brief quotations in a book review.

ISBN: 9798557687621

The goal of this book is to provide helpful information about the complexities of health care in the US. The author and publisher recommend that readers seek advice for specific symptoms or illnesses that require medical supervision. The tips for patients and physicians follow generally accepted public health recommendations. References are provided for informational purposes only and do not constitute endorsement of any websites or other sources. Readers should also be aware that the websites listed in this book may change.

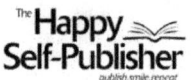

www.happyselfpublisher.com

For Asha

She would have wanted me to write about sickness and suffering.

CONTENTS

Preface xi

PART 1: The Current State of Healthcare in America 1

PART 2: What Patients Need and Want 9

PART 3: What You Should Know About Your Physician and the World That He/She Operates in 39

PART 4: How Outpatient Care is Changing 93

PART 5: The Revolution in Inpatient Care 107

PART 6: Technology: Servant or Master 117

PART 7: First, Do No Harm 125

PART 8: The Journey to Zero Harm 161

PART 9: Tips for Patient Safety 187

PART 10: Tips for Physician Success and Wellness 195

PART 11: The Seven Pillars of Healthcare Reform 201

PART 12: How Servant Leaders are Making a Difference in a Broken Healthcare System 219

Appendix A 225

Appendix B 231

Appendix C 235

Bibliography 239

Acknowledgments 283

PREFACE

The *GOOD OLD DAYS*

I slept and dreamt that life was joy. I awoke and saw that life was service. I acted and behold, service was joy

- Rabindranath Tagore

Things were simpler in the "good old days." Simpler did not necessarily mean better. For example, there were few sophisticated machines, modern hospitals or female physicians. You trusted the family doctor. He was there for you day or night, through snow, storms and sleet. His small black bag carried a stethoscope, a few magic potions and a small hammer. The reusable syringe and needle were disinfected with boiling water. A good diagnostician, he needed few tools. He believed that taking a good history led to a diagnosis 80% of the time. His physical examination skills were superb. The internet, Intensive care units, CT scans and MRIs did not exist. He knew that most common maladies were self-limited, and that most patients get better on their own without medications. His office staff knew you by your first name. You brought gifts, pies and cookies to the office during holidays.

When you were very ill, your doctor admitted you to the hospital and visited again after office hours. Nurses called him as needed. You felt safe. He wrote brief notes with a fountain pen, unburdened by administrative rules and consulted colleagues about your symptoms over a cup of coffee or cigarettes. As the captain of the ship, his number one job was looking out for you. The healing came from the laying of hands, soothing words and sometimes from the scalpel. He was there for you from the womb to the tomb. The physician-patient bond was strong.

There were few regulations, regulators, health insurers, company rules, or any forms or government interference. The doctor had the final word on how long you could stay in the hospital. There was continuity of care. When things went badly, as they sometimes did, the doctor consoled the family with hugs and attended the funeral. He never sent bill collectors to intimidate. An honor system prevailed. Sometimes, items like eggs or live chickens were bartered in lieu of cash. Deals were sealed with handshakes. There was great trust and forgiveness. Litigation was rare. Indeed, there was admiration for how the doctor got things right most of the time. The terms "malpractice" and "burnout" did not exist. There was little anger and much gratitude. Imperfections within this system, such as the problem of physician paternalism as well as unwanted experiments without consent, were tolerated.

For much of the nation, those are now distant memories. Only a few remember the "dinosaurs" who did so much, for so many, with so little. Older patients remember and crave for the personal touch afforded by their family doctor.

Given the massive advances in health care, no one really wants to go back to the Good Old Days. What people pine for is a balance between science, technology and the touch of the human hand, the warmth of a smile. Patients now feel like a number or a bar code. They are identified as customers, clients or consumers, cared for by "providers," strangers whom they do not know. Marcus Welby MD, the fictional television physician, who embodied the very best in clinical practice, is dead. Lest nostalgia overwhelm us, I am reminded by my colleague Dr. Richard Plotzker, that Welby's younger protégé -Dr. Kiley- was "hip enough to ditch the tie and ride a motorcycle. We were in transition even then!"

It begs an important question; how did we get to the present state of discontent?

PART 1

THE CURRENT STATE OF HEALTHCARE IN AMERICA

Without health, life is not life; it is only a state of languor and suffering - an image of death

~Buddha

My wife Asha was diagnosed with a serious illness which ultimately led to her death in 2018. We had good insurance coverage and, as a physician, I was able to contact superb doctors who moved mountains for us. Her final days were peaceful as kind and competent health care workers catered to her needs. Friends and family members rallied to help. My employer was understanding and generous. We were fortunate but millions of Americans do not have the connections we had.

As I reflect on my 50+ year medical career in India, Kenya and the United States, it is *Deja vu* all over again. It is not a surprise that resource poor countries struggle to provide decent care to their citizens. But it should astonish us that the US, the richest and the most technologically advanced nation on the planet, lags almost all wealthy western nations in the quality of the care it provides to its citizens. Health care today consists of a patchwork of individuals, institutions and industries with no cohesive national goal. Health care in some parts of the US reminds me of health care scenes in poor nations. The quality of care in the US varies from superb to substandard and dangerous.

Friends say they can't find a good doctor or get a timely appointment. Office visits, cold and impersonal, feel like business transactions. The hospital, a place of healing, is staffed by strangers who scurry in and out of dirty, noisy and cluttered rooms. Patients complain of delays, bad food, and sagging beds; ignored call lights and harm from mistakes. Marketing experts are often aghast at the mismatch between clinical brilliance and lousy hospitality.

The Medical Industrial Complex (MIC) including pharmaceutical manufacturers, health insurance companies, device makers, pharmacy benefit managers, brokers and middlemen, hospitals and doctors, are often portrayed as the villains in the never-ending spiral of rising costs. The MIC's fiduciary responsibilities to create wealth for themselves or shareholders are understandable but are not well aligned with the goal of improving health. Indeed, some of their practices are blatantly unethical or predatory. Doctors often express revulsion about the economic and emotional harm caused to patients by such practices but they too bear some responsibility for the current disarray.[1]

My fellow health care workers treat millions of the sick and scared with care and compassion each day. However, when we inadvertently hurt someone, a pervading sense of guilt and worthlessness overcomes us. The good we do, gets buried under the overwhelming shame. A lawsuit opens the already festering wound.

Fear of institutional reprisals and litigation silences employees. Little gets reported and even less gets fixed. Hospitals, concerned about their reputation and finances, perpetuate the problem by being less than honest with families or by not acknowledging the human frailties which lead to errors. The tragic incident is quickly forgotten as the next crisis diverts attention from the previous fiasco.

Princeton professors Anne Case and Nobel laureate Angus Deaton, state "It makes good sense for rich countries to spend large amounts to extend their citizens' lives and to reduce pain and suffering.

SICK AND SCARED

But America does it as badly as it is possible to imagine." They ask, "How is it possible that Americans pay so much and get so little? The money is certainly going somewhere. What is waste to a patient is income to a provider."[2, 3]

We hear murmurs about greedy doctors who have abandoned their Hippocratic Oath. When polled for traits of highest honesty and ethics, most Americans rightly choose nurses (85%) followed by engineers (66%), physicians (65%- a drop of 5 percentage points in 10 years), clergy (40%), politicians, and used car salesmen (10%).[4]

But these surveys hide the other side of the equation: The public is woefully unaware of the widespread suffering of physicians who are victims of a messy health care system over which they have no control. The morale of health care workers is at an all time low. The brutal pressures within the workplace are turning many kind and altruistic individuals into angry cynics.

This begins from the outset of their careers. Dr. Pamela Wible, the physician advocate who has led the fight against physician suicide, writes in her book *"Human Rights Violations in Medicine"* that the work conditions of medical students and trainees are so cruel that they violate the 1948 Universal Declaration of Human Rights. The business of caring has hardened many souls.[5]

Half of all doctors meet formal criteria for "Burn Out" on a generally accepted Maslach survey. At least one physician ends his/her life each day, at a rate said to be higher than in any other profession. Cupcakes are served to exhausted doctors on September 17th - Physician Suicide Prevention Day- to alleviate their suffering. The joy of healing others has been stolen from them.

In a relatively new phenomenon, clinicians who can afford it are contemplating premature retirement. Others have become administrators so they can escape the ever-increasing burdens of direct patient care. Half of all medical schools now facilitate such career switches by offering joint medical, business and law degrees. It is the ticket to a corner office with fixed hours, little patient contact and no night calls. Once physicians cross over to the administrative bench, they are viewed as "oppressors" by those still "in the trenches." (Full disclosure: After a half century of providing direct patient care, I too am an administrator).

A business professor suggests that we need far more middle managers including psychologists and human factors experts to make our health system safer.[6, 7] Untrue, say most doctors. Data from the Bureau of Labor and Statistics shows the number of administrators and middle managers has exploded by 3000% in the past four decades (1970-2009). During this period, the number of doctors rose 150%.[8] Critics say "administrators were given Miracle-Gro and doctors got a weed killer."[9] The administrators were brought in to improve efficiency, safety and to reduce costs and waste but can claim little success with any of those objectives.

Many Americans still believe that we get the best health care in the world. That is not the case. Despite high expenditures, the quality of US medical care -using parameters such as life span, infant mortality, and incidence of obesity - ranks number 35 out of 169 advanced economies. USA ranks behind Spain, Italy, Iceland, Japan, Sweden, Switzerland, Australia, Singapore, Norway, Israel, Luxembourg, France, Austria, Netherlands, Canada, S Korea, NZ, Ireland.[10,11] And the US ranks last among nine of the wealthiest nations including Switzerland, Norway, France, Austria, Sweden, Canada, New Zealand, Netherlands, UK, Germany for life expectancy, according to the Commonwealth Fund which is a philanthropy founded by Anna M Harkness in 1918 to "enhance the common good." The average life expectancy in Switzerland is 83.6 years versus 78.6 in the US.[12]

Middle-class families, unable to afford insurance premiums but too "rich" to qualify for state or federal assistance, are seething. In the richest nation on earth, some must choose between medicines, utilities, or putting food on the table. Insurance companies and their brokers seduce people into buying expensive coverage with high deductibles, co-pays and supplemental coinsurance as well as accepting exclusions in coverage. Disjointed approval processes, requirements for preauthorization, penalties for "outside the network" treatment, and surprise bills are the norm. Only half of the US work force is covered by employer paid health care and that does not cover all the costs.

Patients who are unable to pay grossly inflated bills are being sued by hospitals and courts are garnishing their wages.[13] No wealthy country has such a high proportion of uninsured or underinsured citizens. Highly compensated administrators follow merciless rules enacted by Big Money (pharmaceutical companies, pharmacy benefit managers, brokers, middlemen, insurance companies, device manufacturers). Politicians are heavily influenced by lobbyists and huge campaign contributions. It is a giant rip-off. Worse still, crooked doctors steal money from government programs or overcharge patients who obviously cannot afford it.

Health care costs, approaching 20% of the Gross Domestic Product, and more than $11,000.00 per person, are still rising rapidly. Employers are reeling under the burden paying out almost $20,000.00 per worker to get inefficient and wasteful care. Waste in health care has been difficult to define and takes many forms. It may be due to administrative bloat, inefficient delivery of care, overuse of tests, unnecessary interventions, disjointed handoffs, fraud and costs of middlemen. We might even accept the waste within health care - around 30% of our health care dollars- if the care were safe, reliable and effective.

Medical errors result in almost 1000 preventable deaths each day in the US. If these were to be reported on death certificates, they would become the third most common cause of death; just behind heart disease and cancer.[14] Thousands more suffer temporary or permanent harm. Affected patients are rarely told the complete truth about what happened in the hospital or operating room.

Even though the past century has seen amazing progress in Medicine and Science, future generations will laugh at our "primitive" methods, just as we sneered at the practices of a previous generation. Health care will be driven by technology with a focus on accuracy, speed and efficiency. Most of the currently available gadgets and widgets, watches and wearables will be replaced by much better products. In this highly technical world, we may lose the healing power of personal touch, empathy and compassion that patients desperately seek. "The Good Old Days" will never return but perhaps we will find ways to make the physician-patient interaction happier and safer and more deeply satisfactory than it is now. Dr. Eric Topol, a cardiologist, the founder and director of the Scripps Research Translational Institute and a professor at the Scripps Clinic in La Jolla, California, believes we can improve patient- physician relationships by giving the latter what he calls the *"Gift of Time,"* unencumbered by administrative and accounting chores.[15] Most physicians agree that there is insufficient time to take care of needed tasks during patient visits.

Doctors, cynical and angry, feel betrayed. This is not what they signed up for nor what they worked so hard to achieve. Their well-intentioned and motivational dreams about caring and healing have too often become subordinate to administrative chores. Exhausted doctors may appear callous and uncaring, numbed to the fear and suffering of others. Thought leaders are asking whether it is time for us to "organize" and form a national union.[16] to follow the example of The National Union of Residents, boasting 17,000 members, which recently published a list of demands for reform.[17]

The COVID-19 pandemic has taught us that we were woefully unprepared for a national health care crisis. Thousands of lives might have been saved if we had coordinated our responses based on science rather than partisan politics. Amid the bickering and utter lack of leadership, the carnage caused by this virus continues unabated. As I write this, over nine million people have been infected and more than 230,000 are dead at a rate of almost one thousand every day. It has exposed weaknesses at all levels of the health care system. A major overhaul of the entire system is long overdue.

So, what lies ahead for the state of health care? This book explores how we came to this point, what the current realities are and what the future holds for Americans. There are reasons for great optimism and deep concern. My crystal ball, foggy as it is, suggests that there will be seven pillars for change which I will describe in a later chapter. Doing nothing is not an option. Elie Wiesel said:

"What hurts the victim most is not the cruelty of the oppressor, but the silence of the bystander."

I am not an economist, a financial expert, business guru or a policy wonk. I am not famous, and few people know me. However, I have been in health care for over five decades on three continents in disparate health care systems and have firsthand knowledge which others may lack.

My colleagues and I have a passion for our profession and deep compassion for those who are sick and suffering. It is time to change a cruel system, a toxic mix of inefficiency, waste, greed, nepotism, bribery and corruption, which works only for a few, under the guise of free enterprise and capitalism. Hubert Humphrey said, *"Compassion is not weakness, and concern for the unfortunate is not socialism."* Yet, attempts to remedy this can expect considerable opposition.

We have brilliant thought leaders who can help politicians steer this ship safely. We need elected leaders who think about the nation, not rigid ideology, so we can find a win-win situation for everyone. Any reform will be unsuccessful without a partnership with the leaders of the medical-industrial-complex. They have an essential role at the table and to protect the jobs of millions who work in the sectors of the economy they lead.

This book is written for the sick, the scared and for long-ignored clinicians and all health care workers. My goal is to unravel the reasons for the current disarray, to offer tips for patient safety and clinician well-being. The proposed seven pillars of health care reform are aspirational but achievable goals.

The selected stories in this book are actual events retrieved from memory. They represent just a tiny fraction of the errors which harm patients every day. These horror stories, harrowing as they are, must be told. The identities of patients, clinicians and institutions have been omitted, whenever necessary, to protect their privacy.

PART 2

WHAT PATIENTS NEED AND WANT

The good physician treats the disease; the great physician treats the patient who has the disease.

~*William Osler*

The Triple and Quadruple Aims

"The IHI Triple Aim framework" was developed in 2007 by the Institute for Healthcare Improvement[18] in collaboration with others to respond to the crisis in health care. The phrase refers to the simultaneous pursuit of three aims: improving the patient experience of care (satisfaction), improving the health of populations (quality) and reducing the per capita cost of health care (affordability). The aim was broadened to the "Quadruple Aim" after it became obvious that the suffering of clinicians had been excluded.[19]

Sadly, we cannot claim success with any of those goals at this time.

Dr. Stillman and Dr. Tailor wrote about the plight of one man who sought care for abdominal pain. The patient and his wife worked full-time but were too poor to afford insurance and ineligible for Medicaid assistance in Kentucky. The husband had paid a physician a $200.00 fee for an office visit a year earlier for abdominal pain and constipation just to be told he needed further tests which he could not afford. So, he simply used enemas for several months to relieve his severe constipation. Finally, when the pain became unbearable, he went to the Emergency Department (ED) where he was told he had widespread colon cancer. The bill for $10,000 drained his life savings. His wife sobbed as the patient said "If we'd found it sooner, it would have made a difference. But now I am just a dead man walking."[20]

Our health care system failed this family. The authors ask whether it is the obligation of our society, or the individual physician, or both, to take care of the sick to keep them from harm. How would we do that for the millions who have no insurance?

Hubert Humphrey said: *"It was once said that the moral test of government is how that government treats those who are in the dawn of life, the children; those who are in the twilight of life, the elderly; and those who are in the shadows of life, the sick, the needy and the handicapped."*

This quote now rests on the Humbert Humphrey building in Washington DC which appropriately enough, houses the Center for Medicare and Medicaid services (CMS).

Is health care a basic human right?

Americans work long hours, take fewer vacation days than their European counterparts and have a strong sense of justice and fairness. They volunteer in huge numbers to serve the poor and underprivileged and 69% favor universal health care coverage.[21]

But many are afraid that a massive new government program might be even more inefficient, wasteful, than what we have now and that it may take away their right to choose their physician or that it may raise taxes.

Politicians who oppose universal health care proposals label it "socialized medicine" thus aligning themselves with the lobbyists and big businesses which might be harmed by such reform. Many employed Americans with good insurance coverage resent having to subsidize welfare programs including Medicaid, often assuming -incorrectly- that it is the lazy and idle who use it most. They do not welcome the idea of more taxation to support a universal health program. Thus, ideology and individualism has preempted rational discussions about health care, a key to national wellbeing.

Dr. Robert Pearl, a former chief executive within the Kaiser-Permanente Health System, hypothesizes that nations with homogeneous populations, similar culture and appearance, such as Sweden, have a strong sense of community which makes universal health care acceptable. This idea is supported by the rising chorus of opposition to subsidized care in Scandinavian countries as the number of refugees from foreign countries, faiths and cultures rises. Americans are racially, culturally and economically far more diverse and lack that sense of community. Pearl also argues that insured Americans would be more sympathetic if they saw the suffering of the uninsured directly.[22]

Americans have provided for the disabled, the wounded, the elderly and the poor ever since Independence in 1776. Civil war pensions for disabled soldiers and widows, the creation of the Veterans Administration hospital system in 1930, and the passage of the Social Security in 1935, were followed by the Medicare program for those over 65 and the disabled in 1965. These examples of American "socialism" have been widely accepted and welcomed. Most beneficiaries depend on these programs and would be unwilling to give them up. The Affordable Care Act was enacted in 2010 and provided insurance to 30 million uninsured Americans but remains controversial. I have included a more detailed history of Government programs in **Appendix A**.

Why everyone should have a primary care physician (PCP)

A good primary care physician (PCP) is the quarterback in the team. He/she can help prevent chronic illnesses, improve the quality of life, keep economic costs as reasonable as possible, prevent premature death, guide patients when they are ill, and connect them to other experts as needed. The typical primary care doctor is trained in internal medicine, family medicine or pediatrics.

In a study of life-style behaviors, Hecht et al found only 1 in 5 Americans was compliant with guidelines for exercise, good diet, avoidance of cigarettes and excessive alcohol, and a healthy Body Metabolic Index (BMI).[23] In light of this, primary care providers can play a big role as a personal advocate.

Fewer patients are receiving primary care than in previous years. In a large cohort studied by Harvard researchers, primary care visits *decreased* 24% overall among Americans aged 18-64 from 2008-2016 and the percentage of adults who had no primary care *increased* from 38% to 46%. Younger adults were particularly likely to skip primary care visits with the declines being largest for lower income adults. Emergency department (ED) and urgent care center visits on the other hand increased by 47%.[24] The authors speculated that patients were having trouble finding primary care; or were avoiding routine visits due to cost; or went to an urgent care center when they got sick. The authors also wondered whether internet savvy healthy patients were skipping visits for relatively minor illnesses, or they were going to specialists directly. It is possible that patients were skipping "routine follow-up visits" if they felt they were unnecessary.

Access to Primary Care

While it is important to have a PCP, it is increasingly difficult to find one. Estimates of primary physician shortages in the nation range from 21,100 to 55,200. Those positions are increasingly occupied by graduates of osteopathic schools as well as international medical graduates (IMG). Indeed, 68.9% of all IMGs enter primary care fields.[25]

The number of primary care doctors who are now employed by a hospital or a large private practice group has risen from 26% in 2012 to 50% in 2020. This trend has not improved access. Patients seeking a PCP often discover that many private practices are "closed" to new patients. Some practices do not accept Medicare and/or Medicaid because those programs do not pay as well commercial insurers and the care of the elderly, and the socially marginalized, takes more time. Another problem is that the doctor you wish to see may not be in that insurer's network.

I frequently receive phone calls from friends asking if I can help speed up an appointment for them and do try to do so. However, that creates a little guilt since prioritizing my friend's needs may lengthen the waiting period for others. Appointments in private practices and hospital clinics are often weeks or many months away. Ironically, these delays are exactly what opponents of "socialized healthcare" or a universal prepaid system worry about. Elite hospitals, more efficient and keener to increase market share, offer appointments within 2-3 weeks.

Access to the PCP during "off hours" is even more problematic. Horror stories abound about the run around patients suffer. Patients with an urgent question are greeted by receptionists with varying degrees of skill or empathy. The automated message during "off hours" invariably cautions one to "call 911 if it is an emergency" or to go an emergency room. The onus of determining the urgency is passed to the patient. Access for the frail and feeble, hard of hearing, handicapped, visually impaired and for those with language barriers, cognitive impairments or technological challenges is even more difficult and more than 36 million Americans cannot read.[26]

How to choose a primary care clinician

Some prospective patients have an advantage of familiarity with the medical community and its processes, enabling them to secure access more easily. Word-of-mouth, especially from other physicians or nurses, is a good way to initiate a fruitful search. They know who the best doctors are.

Most doctors must take rigorous examinations, usually written multiple choice questions, and surgeons typically must take an oral examination in addition. Once they pass these, they are certified by the Boards of those specialties. Board certification is a reasonable metric for physician selection, and most institutions now insist on such qualifications before granting physicians the privileges to practice. A certificate, of course, does not guarantee good clinical skills, judgment or bedside manner. Recent medical graduates are more likely to be up to date with new developments and more likely to welcome new patients.

Most patients will be treated at some time in their medical journey by a physician trained overseas (International Medical Graduate or IMG) or by a person of color. It can cause anxiety to meet someone with a different cultural or religious background and a different accent. Patients might be assured by the data which clearly shows that a person's race, religion, national origin or where they went to medical school does not affect capability if they have also received training in the US and are board certified. Patient outcomes are no different, and might be slightly better, when patients are cared for by IMGs versus US trained physicians. The reader is directed to APPENDIX B for details about the history of physician immigration to the US since 1965 and their value to the nation.

Choosing a Specialist/Consultant

Specialists do not generally provide primary care. Most specialists still make hospital rounds and have an office practice. But specialists such as dermatologists, rheumatologists and psychiatrists, find it very time consuming -and less lucrative- to visit hospitalized patients. They can see many more patients in the office instead of commuting. By severing connections with the hospital, they also escape its administrative demands to take emergency calls, pay dues, serve on committees, teach without compensation and attend meetings.

As an infectious disease specialist, I was surprised when a colleague told me they are doing the reverse: cutting back on outpatient capacity citing low reimbursement, time consuming work and "frivolous" consultations. They plan to focus on inpatients that need more care and generate higher revenues. The wait time for an office visit to an outpatient infectious disease practice and several other specialties, is now several weeks to months.

Hospitalized patients should ask if they wish to see a specific specialist they know. Otherwise they will be assigned one. Even that is no guarantee that you will get the consultant you chose if he/she is not on call.

Choosing by Gender

Deborah Tannen, a linguistic professor in Washington DC, wrote that women tend to have more face-to-face conversations and make more eye contact than men do.[27] It augurs well for our profession that for the first time in US history, the number of female medical students exceeds the number of male medical students.

Patients may prefer a female clinician for cultural or religious reasons. Additionally, female clinicians are known to be better listeners and spend more time with patients.

A NY Times article reported that mortality rates and readmission rates in a cohort of 580,000 patients with heart disease were lower when female physicians managed the patients compared to those managed by male doctors. Previous studies from Harvard and Johns Hopkins have come to similar conclusions.[28]

Female physicians are more diligent than men in following guidelines and achieving target doses of beta-blockers for patients with heart failure.[29] They achieved better glycemic (sugar) control for diabetics; they prescribe anti-hypertensive medications more often; and they control lipid levels and hypertension better than male physicians do.[30] In a light-hearted piece, Dr. Rada Jones says that not only do female physicians listen and communicate better, but are more thorough, have fewer readmissions, lower heart attack mortality rates, do not wear "germy" ties, are good at multitasking, and have smaller hands for gentler pelvic examinations![31]

Dr. Reinhard Roos, a longtime friend from Munich, Germany echoes some of those feelings, writing: "medicine became female in Germany" because "girls are much better at school than boys" and simply "much smarter than their male counterparts in the medical system." But women have many more responsibilities at home and may choose to work part time. (Personal communication, email dated January 20th, 2020)

Choosing by age

Over 25% of US physicians are older than 65. There is a raging debate about the quality of care provided by older doctors because it is known that cognitive skills and physical stamina decline with age. A recent paper suggests that within the same hospital, patients treated by older general internists and hospitalists (physicians who admit and care for patients only in the hospital), had higher mortality rates than patients cared for by younger physicians. This was only true for older doctors with reduced patient volumes. The thirty-day mortality for patients treated by doctors younger than 40 was 10.8%, 11.1% for doctors aged 40-49, 11.3% for doctors aged 50-59 and 12.1% for physicians older than 60.[32]

What to expect during the physician visit and reasons for patient dissatisfaction

Patients know that doctor visits tend to be short and often unsatisfying. They want a calm, caring and capable physician who will establish eye contact, sit down, listen, display empathy and avoid medical jargon. It is known that patients are interrupted within 18 to 45 seconds by male clinicians while female clinicians tend to listen for an average of 3 minutes before interrupting. In 1984, Drs. Beckman and Frankel studied patient-physician interactions for 74 office visits. They reported that only 23% of patients could complete his or her opening statement. Sixty-nine percent were interrupted by the MD who then directed the conversation. Eight percent of patients were not asked anything![33]

Our communication skills have not improved since 1984. That was the conclusion of two subsequent studies, one conducted in 1999 [34] and the other in 2019.[35] Both concluded that physicians often do not elicit patient concerns, and when they do, they interrupt the patient within seconds. These hasty and incomplete interactions can lead to late-arising clinical concerns and missed opportunities to gather important patient data. Of interest, fellowship trained physicians were more likely to elicit concerns and allow patients to complete their opening statement (44%) than those who were not fellowship trained (22%).

An elderly woman complained that a female physician sat on a "highchair" behind a computer screen, without eye contact, and was invisible except for "the outline of her genital anatomy." The physician was quite surprised - and hurt- because she thought the visit had gone well. The room set-up was changed after this episode. Patients feel neglected when the physician buries his/her face in front of the computer screen and talks while typing. My friend, Dr. Abraham Verghese, has coined the term *iPatient*, to describe such emotional detachment between the patient and the doctor.[36] Clinicians are being forced (by economics and employers) to complete many formalities during a short visit: type or dictate a note, write prescriptions, print patient-education pamphlets and counsel the patient. Many take their work home. A senior internist told me that he never uses the computer when the patient is in the room as a matter of courtesy, and patients love him. But the unfinished work must be done in the evening, at work or at home during what has been called "pajama-time." He does not ask for or get overtime pay. The supervisor may not even be aware. The average pajama time for family physicians is 86 minutes.[37]

The compressed office visits have adverse consequences. A study of interactions between inpatients and physicians was conducted at Yale University. There were significant differences between patients' and physicians' impressions about patient knowledge and inpatient care received. Only 18% of the patients could name their main physician but 67% of physicians thought patients knew their names. Most physicians (77%) believed patients knew their diagnosis; however, only 57% of patients did. Only 58% of patients thought that physicians always explained things in a comprehensible way. Two thirds reported receiving a new medication in the hospital, yet 90% were never told about the adverse effects of these medications. Most physicians (98%) stated that they sometimes discussed their patients' fears and anxieties but 54% of patients said their physicians never did this.[38]

Hospital Consumer Assessment of Healthcare Providers and Systems (HCAHPS)

The HCAHPS survey was developed by The Centers for Medicare & Medicaid Services (CMS) and the Agency for Healthcare Research and Quality (AHRQ). The goal was to survey patients about hospital care. Over 4000 short-term, acute care, non-specialty hospitals participate in the HCAHPS Survey. The survey is administered to a random sample of adult patients across medical conditions between 48 hours and 6 weeks after discharge; the survey is not restricted to Medicare beneficiaries. CMS publicly reports the results on the Medicare.gov-Hospital Compare website four times a year. The survey includes 29 questions related to nurse and physician communication, responsiveness of hospital staff, communication about medicines, discharge information, care transitions, cleanliness, quietness, hospital ratings and willingness to recommend the hospital to others. Doctors and nurses generally get unfavorable reviews for communication from 20-30 % of patients.

Discharge plans

Patients discharged from the hospital are asked to make appointments with doctors, occupational and physical therapists and others within 2-7 days. This can be a huge challenge for patients who have no PCP or if the primary doctor or specialist is not contacted directly by the discharging team. Primary physicians are often unaware that their patient was admitted or that the patient's prescriptions were changed. Endocrinologists cringe when their patients get admitted because the meticulous diabetes control which they had achieved for their patients over years is often upended by these brief admissions. Changed doses and substituted medications are ordered without any discussion with the original prescriber. Worse, the patient then calls the office to say they need to be seen in three days (per instructions from the hospital) when the schedule does not even come close to accommodating that request.

A dangerous omission occurs when the discharge summary does not mention the results of tests which were done or those which are still pending, doses which were changed or drugs which were substituted. Things fall through the cracks all the time because the PCP is rarely kept in the loop. A great hospital will arrange all the appointments for the patient before discharge.

Language barriers

A patient of Burmese descent with limited English Language proficiency was turned away from the MRI suite at Bronson Battle Creek Hospital in Michigan on December 2, 2019 because of difficulty in communication. It is a legal requirement for hospitals to provide interpreter services, but the patient was falsely informed they did not have an interpreter. An employee asked her "Do you even understand what I'm saying to you? Do you know what an iPad is?" A complaint was filed by the family with the hospital and the US Justice Department and Human Health Services. The hospital apologized.[39]

Relatives are not objective interpreters for a variety of reasons. For example, a teenager may withhold information about unmarried sexual activity, pregnancy or symptoms of venereal disease from a parent who might mete out harsh punishment for such revelations. A husband may, based on his personal, religious or cultural preferences, lie to the clinician about his wife's desire for contraception. Most important though is the fact that most family translators are unfamiliar with medical terms, creating the risks of misinterpretation.

Respect and empathy

I took my mother to see a famous orthopedic surgeon for severe arthritis of both knees. The surgeon did not say a word to my sari-clad mother perhaps assuming she was illiterate. A simple hello would have uncovered her fluency in English. The visit lasted one minute with a quick look at the x-rays and a recommendation for a surgical procedure (arthroscopy) which is not effective for such types of arthritis. The procedure did not help and set me back by $10,000. My mother was not pleased and asked for a second opinion. The next surgeon spoke to her directly and explained what he would need to do to make her feel better. He replaced both knees and she was able to walk without pain for many more years.

Patients want a bilateral, un-rushed dialogue, not the caricature of a hand on the doorknob and a foot outside the door. Empathy is fundamental to our craft, and essential for healing. Dr. Thomas Lee, a Harvard cardiologist and the Chief Medical officer at Press Ganey Associates, spoke at a meeting I attended some years ago about his book *An Epidemic of Empathy*.[40] His main message: compassion and empathy for patients is not only the right thing to do but is a good business strategy. Dr. Lee is right, of course, but I felt sad that we needed to be reminded about an attribute which is supposed to be a core ingredient of our profession. His suggestions echo the recommendations by Koster et al that we must make patients our #1 priority as a business strategy to retain their loyalty, and to compete in the marketplace.[41]

Empathy takes time and patience. There is no such thing as "hurry-up empathy." The current economics of medicine permit no more than ten-to-fifteen minutes per patient. If doctors slow down, they get backed up, and this angers those patients who are waiting. The clinician is the hamster on a treadmill who must-see an ever-increasing number of patients to bolster lower revenues and escalating costs while remaining true to his profession. How does one carve out enough time for empathy?

Demetrio Aguila, a Nebraska surgeon, found a novel way. He asks needy uninsured patients to pay for surgery by asking them to volunteer for local humanitarian groups. The volunteer hours are calculated based on the complexity of the surgery. He takes a financial hit, but patients maintain their self-respect and dignity by paying it forward.[42]

Singlism

The word "singlism" was coined by psychologist Bella DePaulo, Ph.D., who is an expert on single people, and author of the book *Singled Out: How Singles Are Stereotyped, Stigmatized, and Ignored, and Still Live Happily Ever After*. She writes: "People who do not have a serious coupled relationship (my definition, for now, of single people) are stereotyped, discriminated against, and treated dismissively. This stigmatization of people who are single - whether divorced, widowed, or ever single - is the twenty-first-century problem that has no name. I'll call it singlism." She says it should be a word in the dictionary.[43]

I was unaware of the effect of singlism in health care until I met Dr. Joan DelFattore, Professor Emerita of English and legal studies at the University of Delaware. She writes about singlism from personal experience. Diagnosed with stage IV gallbladder cancer, with spread to the liver, and a poor prognosis, a surgeon made a bold decision to operate and removed the cancerous tissue. However, one oncologist was unwilling to offer aggressive chemotherapy post-surgery because of her single status assuming she had no support systems. She sought another opinion. That decision saved her life and she is well and active nine years later.[44]

Should patients rely on online reviews of physicians?

Most patients do not write reviews regardless of their true feelings for the doctor. The Intermountain Health System in Utah asked patients to review physicians after each encounter. A sizable number did and were shared with physicians. Many other systems now do that. It allows physicians to correct bad practices and gives patients some objective way to choose their physician. A doctor who consistently gets 5 stars in hundreds of reviews is likely nice and capable. An isolated vicious review is at best unreliable, at worst vindictive and may be untrue.

A bad review may be triggered by events during a visit. A neurologist was extremely upset when someone, in an online review, questioned his credentials, manners and skills. The doctor had apparently discovered he was being recorded surreptitiously and felt he should have been asked for permission. He was angered by the vicious review and sued the patient for defamation, libel and conspiracy to mislead.[45]

Finding a good hospital

Geography generally determines where one gets care. But if you are dissatisfied with your local hospital, CMS has an excellent website (Medicare.gov-Hospital Compare) where hospitals are ranked in 1-5-star categories. The website collects and shares data about hospital safety, efficiency, patient satisfaction, surgical complications and accreditation.[46] Leapfrog and the US News and World Report have different rating systems. Most hospitals guard their reputation very closely and try to put out fires before the news gets in the newspapers or social media. These websites will provide a good starting point. Just make sure the hospital you choose is not "out of network."

Large billboards on highways may show pictures of celebrities endorsing a hospital. It is confusing when there are multiple billboards representing different health care systems in the same town. These advertisements are placed so the brand name becomes familiar to drivers. They have nothing to do with the quality of care you will receive. The celebrities likely don't get their care in that hospital.

Recommendations from friends may help make more informed choices. One can find medical expertise in most large hospitals, but patients are also concerned about efficiency, courtesy, cleanliness or the risk of harm. One clue to efficiency is the speed with which patients are connected to a human being and how quickly you can secure an appointment.

Nonprofit hospitals are exempt from income, property and sales taxes but, in exchange, they are supposed to provide charity and community services. (Charity care is not the same as covering bad debt). I have not seen any data comparing the quality of care of nonprofit versus for-profit hospitals. We do know that for both insured and uninsured patients, nonprofit hospitals that made a lot of money, gave disproportionately less than those hospitals which had lower earnings.[47]

Bills

Hospital bills are inflated, irritating, un-itemized and inaccurate 80% of the time.[48] You will rarely receive a bill which is lower than what you expected. Billing experts advise that everyone, especially those who are self-pay patients, should check the bill carefully for drugs not received, and for services billed for days you were not in the hospital. They advise trying to negotiate 35-50% off the bill. When third parties pay the bill, there is little incentive to scrutinize the charges.

In the real world of commerce, there is often a discount for cash payments. In health care, insurers and hospitals or medical practices negotiate rates which are almost always lower than what an uninsured, self-pay patient is asked to pay. The irony: those who cannot afford health care insurance are asked to pay much more than those who can!

Dozens of unfamiliar health care workers enter patients' rooms several times each day. Patients cannot keep track of who is who. Very few leave a business card. And patients don't get an estimate or a bill at the end of each visit. Every time a health care worker walks into a hospital room, it is generating a charge. It is not like the grocery store where customers know what the milk, tomatoes and cucumbers will cost. All the charges are aggregated at the end of the hospital stay with incomprehensible codes. Bills for nursing care, pharmacy, supplies, doctor visits, physiotherapy, occupational therapy, phlebotomy, lab, consultants, facility fees, iv tubing, bandages, the pill for a headache, for insomnia or for constipation, are all charged. And even the brief physician "visit" -a hand on the doorknob and a foot outside the room- generates a charge. Then there are the "surprise bills" because an "out-of-network" doctor was consulted, and those services are not covered by your insurance plan.

Mind-boggling disparities exist in billing for identical services across the USA. Costs and charges are totally incongruous. A one-dollar item may be billed at $40.00 or even $400.00. CMS recently finalized a price transparency rule which requires hospitals to disclose online the rates they negotiate with insurers for 70 CMS-mandated services and other "shoppable services."[49] The American Hospital Association opposed this plan for financial transparency.

Elizabeth Rosenthal, author of the book *An American Sickness* cites several examples of price-gouging and writes "It may be perfectly legal in health care but would be considered fraudulent in almost every other business."[50] She cites examples of "impostor billing." This occurs when a resident sutures a cut on the finger, but a very high bill comes from the senior surgeon who was not even there; or when the neck collar used for one hour is billed at $319 but costs far less at Walgreen's; or when "the drive- by" visit from a physiotherapist is billed at $646 for a brief encounter; or when the "enforced upgrade" - when a surgeon asks to meet in the ED instead of his office - writes a prescription and charges $1,330. If this prescription had been called in from the surgeon's office, there would have been no charge at all.

A young boy's family received a bill for thousands of dollars when he fell and broke his nose. The injury did not require more than a consultation to the ear, nose and throat specialist but the trauma team had also been consulted. That consultation generated an automatic extra charge of $5000 for a very brief visit. The patient's family appealed. The hospital involved in this episode did a thoughtful review and agreed with the family that the consultation was unnecessary and waived the charge.

Most patients are not so lucky with their appeals. We have become accustomed to this unimaginable financial assault on common sense and decency. Reform will need extraordinary new leaders with courage and integrity.

Affordable medications

Drug costs are hurting Americans. A 2017 national survey revealed that 29% of adults age 19-64 asked the doctor for cheaper medications and either skipped doses, stopped taking the prescription or never filled the prescription. The rates varied from 21.6% in California to 41.9% in Texas.[51]

Frederick Banting and medical student Charles H. Best discovered insulin in the pancreatic extracts of dogs and went on to successfully treating a diabetic dog by injecting it with the extract on July 30, 1921. Soon after, they teamed up with James B. Collip and J.J. R. Mcleod to treat a boy with severe diabetes using a purified product. Banting and Macleod received the Nobel Prize in 1923 and sold the patent to the University of Toronto for one dollar, stating that they had done the work to help sick people, not to get rich. Eli Lilly then won the right to manufacture the drug. Subsequently, others entered the business too. Mass production became possible through recombinant DNA gene technology.[52]

One hundred years later, we have the irony of Americans crossing over into Canada, where insulin was discovered, in order to obtain affordable vials. There is no shortage of insulin in the US. All pharmacies have it. What they don't always have are all the competing brands of rapid and long acting insulin at the same time, and there are laws that prevent them from substituting one brand for another. If the pharmacist called the physician, there might be the possibility of a substitution. But many pharmacists will not take the time to do so. It is shocking that lifesaving medicines can suddenly become unaffordable or inexplicably unavailable because of regulations. Laura Marston tweeted:

One vial a week, keeps me alive; used to cost $20, now it's $275. [53]

Alarmingly, insulin is being sold on Craigslist at discounted prices in an unregulated manner. My colleagues at Christiana Care, led by Jennifer Goldstein MD, MSc, Director Of Clinical Research at The Value Institute at Christiana Care) found 327 ads from sellers who were offering analog insulin products at a fraction of the retail cost. Her team searched all the cities in each state listed on Craigslist between June 12 and June 24, 2019. The average price for analog insulin was about one-tenth of the retail price: $30.24 versus $372.30. The team was particularly worried about storage, potency or contamination. Sellers gave a variety of reasons for wanting to sell: It was leftover by a deceased relative or from a changed prescription. Some sellers professed altruistic reasons including a desire to prevent waste. Some said they were selling because they needed the money for co-pays on newer medications.[54]

The outcry over supply and pricing resulted in Lilly offering the drug at a monthly cost of $35 and CMS doing the same for Medicare recipients through a private-government partnership. This demonstrates that it is possible for government and pharmaceuticals to partner for the common good. And, according to an experienced endocrinologist, "Walmart started a house brand called Relion which is 70/30 human insulin manufactured for them by Novo. It sells for $25 a vial, not in the modern pens. The doctor could be bypassed provided the patient still had syringes. Again, the knowledge of the specialist on how to do this is essential." (Personal Communication from Dr. Richard Plotzker, email dated August 11th, 2020)

In 2017, a businessman with a constant smirk on his face sat in the courtroom listening to charges against him. Martin Shkreli is currently in prison on charges of defrauding investors. But he is more famous for jacking up the price of pyrimethamine, a lifesaving drug for a dangerous infection caused by the parasite toxoplasma, from less than $13.50 per tablet to $750 per tablet (a 5000% increase) while serving as chief executive of Turing Pharmaceuticals. It became an existential crisis for immune-compromised babies and patients with HIV infection.

SICK AND SCARED

Shkreli continued to run his business in prison by using a contraband phone; such was his greed and callousness. He has no medical background but knew that there was no law which forbade him from acquiring a generic drug manufacturer and to charge whatever he wanted for the product. He is now charged by the Federal Trade Commission and the NY attorney general with attempting to block generic competitors from manufacturing pyrimethamine by restricting access to samples and its ingredients.[55]

EpiPen is an injectable vial which patients with severe life-threatening allergies must carry all the time to use in case of an emergency. Moreover, it has a short shelf life and must be renewed frequently. Davis Lazarus, a business analyst for the LA Times, wrote a column on June 5, 2018 about the CEO of Mylan Labs, Heather Bresch, who raised the price of EpiPen injections from $100 to $600 overnight. She expressed no remorse over that decision and blamed it on faults within the health care system, not on company greed. A week after hiking up the cost, her total compensation as CEO soared by nearly 700% — from $2.5 million in 2007 to almost $19 million in 2015, as the drug became more expensive. In an ironic twist, competitors stepped in and the company sales have plummeted. In addition, Mylan finalized a $465 million settlement with the Justice Department for underpayments of rebates to Medicaid programs.[56]

Tamiflu is a drug recommended for severe influenza and is routinely prescribed for seriously ill or elderly patients. A whistle blower, Thomas Jefferson MD, has alleged that Roche misled the US and local governments into stockpiling $1.5 billion worth of Tamiflu for any future flu epidemic by claiming that the drug stopped contagion between people.[57] Many physicians were also brainwashed into believing that contagiousness might be reduced. The truth is that Tamiflu slightly reduces symptoms and attenuates the illness by about 24 hours but does not halt virus transmission between people. As an infectious disease specialist, it has never made sense to me that we prescribe Tamiflu to healthy people with mild flu illness.

An expert panel in the Veterans Administration (VA) determines the best and lowest-priced drugs within a category of generic drugs, thus prompting competition. Medicare is not permitted to do that. It is possible to reduce costs immediately by allowing Medicare to do the same- negotiate better deals for pharmaceutical agents by setting limits on unreasonable price gouging. Medicare could have saved $14.4 billion from an estimated $32.5 billion budget if it used VA-negotiated prices for the 50 costliest Medicare Part D drugs. The cost savings for 31 insulin products in 2017 would have been $3.4 billion out of the $7.8 billion Medicare spent on insulin.[58]

Pharmaceutical companies continue to raise prices citing the cost of drug development and research. The claims that it costs one billion dollars to market a viable drug are almost certainly highly inflated. They correctly claim that theirs is a risky business since most investigational drugs do not reach the market. However, pharmaceutical company profits are almost twice as high as those of other companies on the S&P 500 index.[59] The marketing budgets of the major companies far exceed the budgets for research and development of new products.

Campaign contributions by pharmaceutical, device manufacturers and lobbyists control the political process. Astonishingly, thirty nine of the forty politicians -twenty senators and twenty house representatives- who sit on committees with jurisdiction over these industries have a clear conflict of interest. [60] Contributions peaked during years when there were referendums on drug pricing and regulation. Drug cost reform is likely a long way off without some oversight of such committees.

Credit card debt and bankruptcies

Two thirds of patients said they had to use a credit card to pay a medical bill in 2019 and 10% owed at least $10,000 with interest rates in the 15-20% range.[61] Estimates of bankruptcies caused by health care debts range from 4% to over 60%, the latter number published by a team including Senator Elizabeth Warren when she was a professor at the Harvard Law School. The bankruptcies are likely caused by multiple factors including a loss of income during illness rather than medical bills alone. But even 4% is large number if used as the "floor" for estimates.[62]

Waste

Waste in health care is related to administrative bloat, inefficient delivery of care, overuse of tests, unnecessary interventions, duplication, disjointed handoffs, fraud or the costs of middlemen.

Administrative spending for health care varies greatly between the US and Canada and the gap is widening. It reflects the inefficiencies of the U.S. private insurance–based, multi-payer system. U.S insurers and providers spent $3 trillion on health care of which $812 billion was spent on administration amounting to $2497 per capita or 34.2% of total national health expenditures versus just $551 per capita (17%) in Canada, $844 versus $146 on insurers' overhead; $933 versus $196 for hospital administration; $255 versus $123 for nursing home, home care, and hospice administration; and $465 versus $87 for physicians' insurance related costs.[63] Shrank et al estimated the cost of waste to be around 25% ($760-$935 billion) of total health care spending in the US and that there was a potential to eliminate at least one-fourth of this waste.[64]

Donald Berwick, a distinguished leader in the safety movement, asks "Is waste marbled so thoroughly into health care processes and structures that no scalpel is fine enough to work it free?" The report by Shrank, he says, finds the opposite; that there are indeed ways to cut waste.[65]

Medicare- the "socialistic" program- has much lower administrative overheads (<3 %) but fraud by physicians, con-men, suppliers and pharmaceutical companies accounts for almost $60 billion annually.

Pain, Addiction and Suffering

Thresholds for pain vary greatly. Physicians may inadvertently minimize the intensity of discomfort the patient feels leading to under-treatment. To remedy this situation, the Joint Commission created a new standard in 2001 for pain assessment and called it the 5th vital sign, of equal importance to the previous four (temperature, pulse, blood pressure and respiratory rate). A pain scale of 0-10 was developed with a smiley face for zero pain and a frown at the other end. We were told not to question the patient's motives and assured by experts that patients with "genuine pain" did not get addicted. We parroted these lines faithfully. Physicians who withheld narcotics were accused of lacking empathy and being paternalistic. This bandwagon of mercy, the latest fad, moved narcotics rapidly through the health care system. Palliative care specialists and oncologists certainly alleviated much pain and suffering in terminally ill patients, but surgeons routinely gave patients more narcotics than necessary for post-operative pain.

We created a new generation of addicts and then vilified the victims. In 2004, the Joint Commission removed its pain standard because of mounting concerns about a dramatic rise in prescriptions, addiction, a growing black market and overdose-related deaths. But by then the die was set already.

My colleague, Dr. Terry Horton, Chief of Addiction Medicine at Christiana Care and nationally known for his work with Project Engage, describes the agony of addicts as a "primal misery," a desperate craving. Reason and fear desert them as they begin "shopping" around for pills for personal use or for resale in the black market. Some resort to robbery or prostitution, the use of dirty needles, resulting in the spreading of deadly infectious diseases such as HIV and hepatitis C. We began to see a deluge of patients with severe bacterial infections of the spine, bones, flesh, heart valves, brain and other vital organs; which required prolonged treatment under supervision. Costs rose exponentially. Horton adds: "The unfortunate inference many people make is that addiction is a hedonistic endeavor that reinforces for some a moralistic perspective and stigma……The brain learns quickly that this form of primal misery can be rapidly alleviated through use. Use behaviors are repeatedly reinforced. Eventually, even the anticipation of withdrawal engages core motivational circuits to perpetuate drug use. In a sense, primitive pathways, preserved in mankind to avoid pain and suffering are the basis of the disease state." (Personal communication, email dated July 29th, 2020)

Hospitalized patients, often in withdrawal, demand narcotic injections and abuse staff when they do not get their fix in a timely fashion. Friends bring illicit drugs which are injected in hospital bathrooms. Many patients sign themselves out. Some overdose and die. The cost to the nation goes beyond dollars. Young lives are wasted. Families are shattered. In 2019, one young person died each day from an overdose in Delaware, a state with less than one million residents. The number was four times higher in Philadelphia. The crisis caused a decline in the overall life expectancy of Americans and claimed the lives of nearly 450,000 people between 1999 and 2018.

Unscrupulous doctors, teaming up with other crooks, opened pill mills. "Clinics" in strip malls, shops, laundries, and pizza places became fronts for the illicit drug trade. On December 17, 2019, a local physician in Delaware was convicted of prescribing 7,000 oxycodone pills to five people who had no indication for it. The drugs were resold at exorbitant prices.

Purdue Pharmaceuticals was sued by 48 states for aggressively promoting the broad use of Oxycontin, by minimizing the risks of addiction, falsely claiming benefits and encouraging higher doses. Negotiations have broken down towards a $12 billion deal with several states and cities because some members of the Sackler family, which holds a controlling interest in Purdue Pharma, have refused to contribute more to the proposed agreement. The settlement money was to be used to promote the welfare of victims, to help provide antidotes to overdoses, and to support programs to reduce the risk of opioids. Meanwhile, the company has filed for bankruptcy thus halting 2,600 lawsuits brought by cities, counties, states, hospitals and other plaintiffs.

Family members moved at least $1 billion to offshore banks.[66] Purdue recently pled guilty and settled for $8 billion.

Meanwhile, efforts to set up facilities for supervised injections of narcotics, a model which is successful in some European nations, has met great resistance in the US. A clinic proposed by Philadelphia officials would have been the first in the nation to model what the Europeans do. But it never opened because of opposition from the community. An opportunity was lost to explore the potential of such clinics to reduce the primal misery, overdose deaths, crime, imprisonment, broken families and spread of HIV and hepatitis by trying this approach. Addicts could return to work and pay taxes. Illegal importation of drugs by cartels might be thwarted if we provided the drug legally under strict supervision. Drug related crime would go down.

The Tyranny of Employers and Insurers

Insurers have a tight grip on the nation's health. Lauren Bard, an ER nurse, delivered a premature baby on September 18, 2018 at the Irvine Medical Center, California. The tiny baby weighed less than two pounds and had a stormy course with many complications. Irvine's billing department and Anthem Blue Cross had assured her she was covered. However, her plan with the Dignity Health System required enrollment of the newborn within 31 days of birth, something she did not know. The bill was $898,984.57. Eight days past the deadline, she discovered that her baby was not covered by a system which has $6.6 billion in assets and where the CEO makes $11.9 million annually and a dozen or more executives make $1 million or more. If she paid $100.00 each month, it would take her 748 years to pay the entire bill. She appealed to Dignity twice and was turned down. She postponed her wedding so her boyfriend would not get saddled with debts. She considered bankruptcy. All this happened because, as Dignity pointed out, "she should have read the provisions of her policy." She posted this on Facebook on October 7, 2018. ProPublica contacted Dignity, which immediately apologized and reversed its position. Imagine her anguish.⁶⁷ It is perhaps the rule, rather than an exception, that people will not read the fine print either because they trust the system, or the fine print is too small to read, or because they have no choice but to sign papers issued by an insurer who has a contract with the health system.

A Bill to Remember

Dr. Roya Fathollahi, an internist at Manhattan Specialty Care, obtained a throat swab when Alexa Kasdan, a 40-year-old policy consultant, complained of a sore throat and prescribed an antibiotic. The sample was sent to a lab for bacterial and viral cultures as well as sophisticated DNA tests to identify viruses. In my 50 years of clinical practice, I have never seen anyone order such tests for a sore throat. The bill was $28,395.50, most of which was covered by Blue Cross Blue Shield of Minnesota, but the patient was still responsible for more than $2,000.⁶⁸ Such visits are typically brief, and costs should not exceed $100.00. Patients have a right to appropriate services at a reasonable cost.

An Elaborate Hoax

Elizabeth Holmes, the founder of Theranos, was a 19-year-old Stanford dropout whose basic premise was that hundreds of lab tests could be performed from just a few drops of blood on equipment called Edison. Venture capitalists poured money into the project and influential figures like Henry Kissinger, George Schultz, James Mattis and Larry Ellison backed her. However, the tests were being done on machines used by conventional labs because Edison provided inaccurate results. This hoax also fooled the FDA which had approved the technology. Her worth dropped from $9 billion to zero. She and her Chief Operating Officer Ramesh Balwani face 20 years in prison. Her lawyers plan to plead a mental illness at the trial.⁶⁹

How "Observation status" (OBS) ruins families

Hospital stays are expensive. In order to control those costs, CMS introduced "observation status" rules to prevent unnecessary admissions for patients who need brief periods of observation in the hospital. Among the provisions are the following: (a) Observation patients are treated as outpatients with a typical hospital stay of less than 48 hours but with cost sharing (b) Medicare patients who have part A (hospitalization) but not part B (outpatient) are responsible for the entire OBS bill. If the patient needs observation beyond two midnights, they are converted to "admit" status. This is very important for patients to understand.

A patient in OBS status must pay out of pocket if there is a need for further care in a rehabilitation facility unless they were *admitted* for at least three days. Patients often assume that since they were in the hospital, in a bed, and were getting the same care as others, they are "covered." Hence it is critical to ask, "Am I being admitted as an inpatient or under observation status? Will my nursing home costs be covered if I need to go there?"

Jennifer Goldstein MD, MSc (a hospitalist and Director of Clinical Research at the Christiana Care Value Institute, who reported the sale of insulin on Craigslist), and her colleagues studied the effects of OBS on families. They found that low income populations, with a higher burden of disease and thus most vulnerable to repeat admissions, were more likely to incur liability from the costs of the observation rule.[70]

Physicians, unaware of these rules, have been caught in this trap too. A radiologist was shocked when he was hit with a bill for thousands of dollars after surgery for prostate cancer and a hospital bed stay in OBS status.[71]

Burdens of Caregivers

Friends and family members, who provide care for loved ones at home, work just as hard as nurses do. The emotional toll and the financial consequences are underappreciated by society and government. These caregivers are doing backbreaking work. That it is done out of duty and love does not reduce the magnitude of suffering.

Seventy-eight percent of caregivers have out of pocket costs in the $7-12 thousand dollar range. Their retirement savings are reduced by 25%; and 20% take on more debt. One-third cut back on household maintenance and/or on clothing, and the same number have left a job due to the demands of caregiving. Those who continue to work put in 80 minutes less per day. One tenth of all caregivers cut down on children's education or on utilities. Caregivers sleep less and skip their own dental or other care 30% of the time, including postponing tests and prescriptions.[72] They may become irritable and resentful especially if other family members do not pitch in. This boiling cauldron can occasionally lead to elder abuse.

The CARE Act (Care Advise Record Enable), passed by 43 states, requires hospitals to identify a family caregiver in the chart. It is unclear how the act would apply to individuals who have no family but instead rely on friends for support. The caregiver must be notified of a pending discharge and be provided instructions in person. How well it is implemented is unclear. But the act in no way mitigates the suffering of care givers. Society must find a way to reduce the burdens of these silent workers.

Access to Records

The medical record belongs to the patient. CMS launched a national program in 2011 to speed up the use of electronic medical records (EMRs) by patients. And in 2016, they required hospitals to provide digital access to all patients. Well-informed patients can participate in their own health by being aware of what the medical teams are thinking, saying, planning or doing. Some chart notes are inaccurate, misleading or offensive. This program was intended to be an opportunity to inform and correct the record in real time.

So, it was surprising to learn that during the 2014-2016 periods, when 95% of patients in 2410 hospitals had access to their personal record, only 10% looked at it.[73]

The authors noted a digital divide based on predictable socio-economic factors and insurance status. Hospitals and offices often make patients jump through hoops to access their own record. Others offer what is called an "open chart" where patients can view their record online in real time.

Care coordination

It seems logical that primary care doctors and consultants should share their thoughts about complex patients with each other. The tumor board in oncology is an outstanding model for such interactions but it is not routine practice for other disciplines. Reasons given are that it is very time-consuming and hard to schedule meetings. Given the importance of such dialogue, one would think we could overcome the technical bumps; but far too often, physician convenience trumps safety.

Dr. Santina Wheat, a family physician described how she had to use her "MD" status to get things done when her mother was admitted to a hospital. She wondered how people who have no clout or connections get the care they need. She wrote both of pride for her profession as well as fear of the health care system and her struggles, as she tried to get decent care for her mother.[74]

A Commonwealth Fund survey of 13,000 physicians in 11 countries shows the US trails several industrial nations in care coordination with other clinicians, home services and social services despite possessing the most advanced health information technology systems in the world. For example, home visit coordination occurred for only 37% cases in the US vs 70% elsewhere; coordination with other doctors was 49% vs 70%; the ED called primary care doctors 50% of the time vs 80%; social services were called by doctors 40% vs 74%

elsewhere; exchange of patient records between physicians occurred 50% of the time vs 80% (in New Zealand, Netherlands and Norway).[75]

People are harmed when communication is absent. It should not surprise anyone that the US ranks lower than other industrialized nations in most quality measures.

Safety in the hospital

Patients are frightened by rumors and reports of harm due to human errors. A report from the Institute of Medicine (IOM) in 1999 called for action regarding patient safety,[76,] but two decades later, the data suggests we are doing far worse.[14] The number of people killed in American hospitals each day is equivalent to 2-4 jumbo jets crashing daily. Thousands more are maimed.

Airlines take safety much more seriously than hospitals because their planes can be grounded for safety violations. Hospitals do not shut down because they are essential services. In March 2019, the Boeing 737 MAX passenger airliner was grounded worldwide after 346 people died in two crashes, Lion Air Flight 610 on October 29, 2018 and Ethiopian Airlines Flight 302 on March 10, 2019. The year prior to that there were fewer than 100 deaths from airline crashes worldwide. Patients have good reason to fear dangers within hospitals. This topic is examined in more depth in part 7 titled "First, do no harm."

Truth and Lies

Physicians whose mistakes harm patients become "second victims." They want to apologize but the fear of lawsuits, loss of reputation and pressure from their practice partners and hospitals holds them back. Often, they are coached by lawyers, risk managers and other stake holders to remain silent. That reticence is understandable especially when the facts of the case are still unclear. However, the silence is inexcusable when the goal is simply to suppress the facts. Thus, the truth may not be disclosed in a timely manner, if at all. Truth delayed is truth denied. The rehearsed and choreographed product appears insincere. Thought leaders have questioned whether disclosures in a hospital setting can ever be free of institutional constraints or bias and whether they truly make a difference in litigation or forgiveness.[77] But that is irrelevant. The apology makes both sides feel better. We must tell the truth even if it has personal or institutional repercussions.

A team at the Louisville VA hospital in Kentucky reported in 1987 that a sincere apology and complete disclosure of errors had a healing effect on patients and physicians alike. The words "I am sorry" led to decreases in lawsuits and the amount of settlements. I remember making such disclosures to families with full organizational support at the VA hospital where I worked. This concept was largely unknown or ignored in the private sector. The difference may be that VA physicians are not sued individually under the Tort act and may not fear huge settlements or lawsuits as much.[78]

Dr. Allen Kachalia and his colleagues who did extensive work on patient harm and mitigation strategies, also reported that keeping patients and families informed went a long way to reduce lawsuits and the size of settlements, thus supporting the VA initiative.[79]

Dr. Timothy McDonald, when he was an anesthesiologist at the University of Illinois in Chicago, proposed seven pillars for "optimal communication."[80] That morphed into the CANDOR (Communication and Optimal Resolution) program launched by the Agency for Healthcare Research and Quality (AHRQ) in 2015 with grants to a consortium of three health care systems—Christiana Care, the Dignity Health system and MedStar—representing 14 hospitals. I was fortunate to be one of a core group of individuals trained by McDonald and other experts in the field as CANDOR champions to manage similar programs at our own hospitals. Most hospitals in the nation, however, have no formal disclosure programs.

***

In this section, the discussion revolved around what patients need and want. However, patients also need to understand the world in which their doctor operates. That is the subject of the next section.

PART 3

WHAT YOU SHOULD KNOW ABOUT YOUR PHYSICIAN AND THE WORLD THAT HE/SHE OPERATES IN

The philosophies of one age have become the absurdities of the next, and the foolishness of yesterday has become the wisdom of tomorrow.

~*William Osler*

Dr. Robert Laskowski M.D., M.B.A., when he was CEO of the Christiana Care Health system (2003-2014) in Delaware, called for a transformation of health care by "making it easier and better." The words resonated because life has become difficult for both patients and doctors. Both groups are dissatisfied.

A snapshot

The Doctors Company, the largest malpractice insurance company owned by physicians, with 79,000 members asked 3,400 doctors for their opinion about the future of health care. A majority (70%) said they would not recommend Medicine as a profession to others. Even though the average age of the men was only 62 and for women 55, 44% said they were likely to retire in 5 years. More than 50% stated there was a negative impact on their relationships with patients, efficiency and income, and 60% felt their income would decrease under the "value-based model." Of those who wished to continue working, more than 75% want to remain solo practitioners.[81]

The public is unaware of the fury of doctors who blame hospital administrators, insurance companies, government and regulatory agencies for their woes. Doctors who work on the front lines of health care ("the trenches") do not trust or like administrators who hide in badge entry only "fortresses" labeled C-suites. The analogy to battle fields is unfortunate but apt. There is little trust and much mudslinging. Doctors feel they have lost their voice and have no other weapons. Leaders, tired of constant criticism, exclude doctors from their conversations. Curiously, many in the trenches yearn to become administrators to enjoy the same perks -high income, no calls, no patient contact, a corner office with a window and fixed working hours- of high office.

Somehow, the joy of healing others has been stolen from us. This is reflected in many online blogs and conversations such as found on Kevin MD, Doximity, and Sermo.com all with different levels of screening for inflammatory remarks. These blogs are reflective, thoughtful and a window to what physicians are thinking and saying. How did we get to this point of cynicism and anger?

The Electronic Medical Record (EMR)

The EMR makes us miserable. It is the single most important reason cited for physician discontent.

Massive paper charts held thousands of stained and worn or torn pages containing illegible words of wisdom -or gibberish- in varying shades of black and blue ink. The spines holding the chart together cracked and crumbled. Over time, the crumpled dry pages fell out. Sometimes, the unwieldy chart fell to the floor with a thud, broke open and the pages had to be reassembled in chronologic order. Doctors, nurses, students, therapists and anyone who needed to write a note- waited in line to get access, so their words could be immortalized.

People left a fingerprint, pathogens from unwashed hands and crumbs of food or coffee stains on the pages.

The chart traveled with the patient for tests, procedures and appointments within the hospital. When the chart got too heavy, it was retired to a remote, moldy warehouse or basement, where, over time, the pages yellowed, dried up and crumbled. After some years they were destroyed. More modern institutions archived them in microfiche. Sometimes, the old chart simply disappeared forever.

The electronic medical record was supposed to solve the problems of legibility, portability, remote and simultaneous access. Enormous amounts of data could be archived for eternity in an electronic cloud. There was hope that improved legibility and interoperability between computers would improve communication and patient safety. That did not happen.

EMR in the Veterans Administration (VA) system

The VA, with its vast health care network, had introduced EMRs in all VA hospitals by 1999. The software was freely available to any hospital that wanted it. A seamless transition from paper to the EMR occurred seemingly overnight in a VA hospital where I worked. The legible notes, printed prescriptions and medical alerts reduced errors and enhanced patient safety. Communication improved. We could access a patient's chart from VA hospitals across the country. Importantly, our notes were short and precise since they were not tied to billing.

Storage of x-ray images within the EMR came later for most VA hospitals but had been in use at the Washington VA medical center since 1990. We no longer needed to trudge down to the radiology suite, find a film and then request the constantly interrupted and annoyed radiologist to read them for us. Physicians could now review films remotely, from their own offices or homes. There was no need to recycle films to extract the silver.

In 2003, I left the VA system to join a private practice in the same town. This office, like most other private offices and the region's 1000 bed hospital complex (with over 1500 doctors and thousands of nurses) still maintained paper records, not emerging from that medieval age for several more years.

EMR in private hospitals

Cerner and Epic EMR platforms were -and remain- the most popular platforms used by hospital systems. The implementation of Cerner at my private hospital was cautious, stepwise and piecemeal. Initially, the EMR was limited to certain departments and units and included just the history and physical (H&P) and the discharge (DC) summary. Doctor's orders, progress notes, laboratory and radiology reports, vital signs and consent forms remained on paper. Radiology films were not incorporated in to the EMR until much later. Thus, one had to assemble critical information from multiple sites. The intensive care units (ICU) and outpatient offices used systems incompatible with Cerner. Eventually the systems were aligned, but the process was disruptive, and it took many years to complete.

However, the hope that private EMRs across the nation would "talk to each other" (interoperability) never materialized. It also became obvious that the systems, designed without significant clinician input, were geared towards billing and codes rather than towards smooth workflows or physician convenience. The EMR now took much time away for administrative chores at the expense of direct face to face doctor-patient interactions.

EMR in private doctor offices

Private medical offices acquired an EMR around 2011 after the federal government provided financial incentives- $44,000.00 per physician- if the machines fulfilled criteria for "meaningful use," a term very few understood. The idea was part of an effort to improve interconnectivity between offices and hospitals.

Remarkably, incomes in some practices increased significantly even as the workload remained unchanged. Was it due to previous under-coding or the disturbing possibility that the templates, which magically auto-filled a whole paragraph or page with just one click, were resulting in over-coding and over-billing?

The office EMR was, unfortunately, not compatible with the hospital system. That led to the wasteful printing and faxing of paper documents and the risk of violating patient privacy under the Health Insurance Portability and Accountability Act of 1996 (HIPAA). An advanced system called DHIN (Delaware Health Information Network), the first such system in the state, was developed to centralize and share office notes, laboratory reports and hospital data, but it did not provide real-time updates.

The office EMR was one reason I left office practice in 2012 and contemplated retirement. The machine dominated our lives. Billing determined productivity and entitlement to bonuses. The temptation to over-click was ever present. The notes were no longer useful and wasted time. The "charting" detracted from direct patient care.

The Ritual of Documentation and Erosion of Medical Education

Physicians feverishly pound keyboards hoping that each click will enhance the wellbeing of their patients. "Charting"- documenting everything- is time-consuming and results in fewer minutes spent with the patient. The patient's questions, and requests for more detail, have become an inconvenient intrusion in our duty to perform an electronic ritual. It is a brutal race against the relentless clock.

Patients understandably slam doctors for impersonal and rushed visits complaining that "he/she did not even touch me" and sometimes, "did not even look at me." They do not know that the EMR's cumbersome rules keep doctors from doing their job well; from going home, getting enough sleep or enjoying some time off. Atul Gawande, a surgeon at Harvard, in an essay titled "Why doctors hate their computers" describes how a system which was supposed to make things "greener, faster and better" ended up taking up too much time and led to burnout, depression and suicidal thoughts. It was not built for patients or doctors, but for billing and compliance personnel."[82]

He writes "…but three years later I've come to feel that a system that promised to increase my mastery over my work has, instead, increased my work's mastery over me. I'm not the only one." A 2016 study found that physicians spent about two hours doing computer work for every hour spent face to face with a patient—whatever the brand of medical software. Gawande met administrative staff who said that the tasks such as order entry and computer requisitions that they used to perform previously, have been passed on to doctors. The loss of time to attend to patients led to the hiring of scribes or use of virtual scribes. Layers upon layers of administrative chores took time away from patients who began to resent the impersonal care.

Dr. Ranjana Srinivasan, an oncologist and Fulbright scholar at Monash University in Australia, bemoans the replacement of the long-gone fountain pen by an electronic record. The pen recorded the most important items from the visit. The EMR template leaves no personal imprint since one note looks like any other. She wrote. "There was no backspace or delete button, no drop-down menu, no cut and paste — my notes were the best of me wanting the best for my patients."[83]

It has been said that "proper interpretation and use of computerized data will depend as much on wise doctors as any source of data in the past."[84] Verghese et al, commenting on the need for synergy between human touch and technology quotes Francis Peabody's maxim that "….the secret of the care of the patient, is in caring for the patient."[85]

The demands of the machine take away the time to conduct proper interviews and examinations. We are rapidly losing our clinical skills and our ability to think things through. The time for calm reflection has been replaced by thoughtless, reflex actions such as over-prescribing, over-ordering tests and referrals. Standard templates, which are designed to maximize bills, have not been individualized for each practice or specialty or to avoid unnecessary or improper documentation.

Perhaps one of the biggest sacrifices in minimizing in-person time with a patient is the loss of the opportunity to read non-verbal cues of a patient's body language, where more is often communicated than it is in words. My friend, Chuck Selvaggio, the executive director of Neighbors to Nicaragua Inc., says "an evasive turn of the head, a downcast eye, a bursting out into tears, or an uncontainable smile may provide incredibly accurate, helpful information. You can't see any of this if your head is buried in a computer screen."

Not only does the EMR keep us away from patients but it has also eroded the physical examination skills of residents as they learn that technology can replace the bedside examination skills. In an alarming report, researchers described the inadequacies of the physical examination as a cause of medical errors and adverse events. In the 208 clinical vignettes they reported, a physical examination was not done 63% of the time. In 14% of the vignettes, the physical sign was elicited but misinterpreted and 11% missed the relevant sign. The missed findings resulted in delayed, missed, or incorrect diagnosis, unnecessary treatment, unnecessary use of contrast, waste of money and complications. The authors concluded "Physical Examination inadequacies are a preventable source of medical error, and adverse events are caused mostly by failure to perform the relevant examination."[86]

Obtaining a history and doing a bedside examination which, in the past, were enriching and rewarding educational experiences, are now truncated affairs. Most attending physicians, who used to find teaching medical students and residents a mutually beneficial experience, are now reluctant to take on added responsibilities. Teachers of bedside medicine are a dying breed. Increasingly, residents are learning from each other and have little contact with senior clinicians with wisdom, experience and knowledge. Worse, the residents might be learning and teaching bad habits.

Dr. Christine Sinsky's team reviewed the work of 57 physicians in an ambulatory practice in four states for four specialties and found that physicians spend 27% of their total time on direct face to face time with patients and 49.2% on the EMR and desk work. In the exam room with patients, they spent 52% of the time with patients and 37% on the EMR. Those who kept a diary also reported working an extra 1-2 hours at night to catch up.[87]

A study of 2,191 health care organizations, 100 million patient encounters and 155,000 non- surgeons was conducted by Overhage and McCallie from the Cerner Corporation. They reported that on average, physicians spend 16 minutes and 14 seconds for each patient encounter using EMRs and 11% of that time was after hours. Chart review, documentation and writing orders took 33%, 24% and 17% of the time respectively.[88] Clinicians MUST have more time for direct interactions with patients.

No one could have predicted how the EMR would hurt our profession and force us to stray from our mission of patient care.

Templates and Temptation

I met a 93-year-old woman in the office for a brief follow up visit for a toe ulcer. She was examined a week earlier by another physician whose chart note indicated he had done a head to toe examination including a search for lumps in the breasts. This was so improbable that I assumed it was due to an inadvertent click in one box which populated the entire note with predetermined text. Such checklists are being used routinely. One cannot tell whether it is a deliberate attempt to overbill or an oversight. A diligent doctor will edit the note to exclude items which were not performed and add items which are not in the template. I have great concerns about these electronic clicks. Bad habits often become acceptable and permanent.

Dr. Skolnik and Dr. Notte were surprised to read a note by a urologist which mentioned "whispering pectoriloquy," which is a unique sound sometimes heard during a lung examination. Not many physicians know what whispering pectoriloquy is, and fewer still check for it. It is virtually certain that no urologist would perform such an examination. Thus, the authors felt that the "authenticity of the entire note fell in doubt." They were charitable in blaming the design of the EMR for the problem.[89]

Dr. Jay Kostman, a well-known infectious disease clinician in Philadelphia, became a victim of the template (and neglect) when he went to a nearby ED for the sudden onset of leg pain, fever and a headache. He was assured all was well and discharged with no specific diagnosis. Feeling uneasy, he decided to listen to his own heart after he got home and heard a new and loud heart murmur. He self-diagnosed an infection of a heart valve which had caused an infected clot to travel from the heart to his leg and brain and would have been fatal without treatment. He required prolonged antibiotics, surgery for a brain aneurysm and treatment for the clots. The ED physician had, without doing the examination, clicked a template.[90] If physicians cannot trust each other's opinions, how can patients trust us? Was the ED doctor lazy, too busy and overwhelmed, distracted, forgetful or simply habituated to clicking the template for all patients? And even if he had listened to the heart, how can anyone be certain that he/she had the skills to identify the heart murmur?

Cut and Paste

Clinicians often "cut and paste" their own progress note from a previous day and then edit it. This saves time but all the daily notes begin to look alike; page after page of electronic monotony. Clinicians have little time to read so many almost identical notes and may miss vital information.

More egregious is the practice where some physicians simply copy notes written by others and paste them into their own notes without attribution. This makes it appear as though the person had performed their own history or physical examination. This is plagiarism, plain and simple. Chart notes meant to enhance the patient's care have degenerated into a revenue-gathering tool. Some hospitals, using the despised relative value unit method (RVUs) to measure productivity, focus on volume, revenue and documentation, rather than the value of that visit for the patient's health.

Abuse of Remote Access

Remote access to hospital records allows us to review chart notes, read x-rays, provide urgent consultations or type and fax a prescription from the comfort of the office or home. But the privilege can be exploited for personal convenience or revenue and jeopardize patient safety.

A nurse practitioner visit can be billed at 85% of the physician fee. However, if the doctor signs the note (and thereby attesting they have examined the patient) the patient can be billed at 100%. Some physicians and surgeons simply sign all notes remotely without ever touching the patient. That is illegal.

Safety regulations require that patient histories and physical examinations done in an office visit be updated within 30 days of planned surgery to make sure nothing has changed. Too often this update is done minutes before surgery. I am aware of an individual who updated a history remotely, on behalf of his supervising surgeon, while on vacation in another state! This is a dangerous violation of safety rules as well as legal and ethical standards.

Ergonomics

A young Indian professor with a PhD in Ergonomics once told me that his job prospects in India were close to zero because, in his words "There is no value for life, much less for ergonomics. No one cares."

Proper posture and placement of computers and keyboards helps alleviate some of the stiffness as well as the wrist, back, shoulder and neck pain associated with prolonged sitting. In an increasingly sedentary society, ergonomics is an important part of wellbeing.

India is not alone. In my 50 years in the US, I have never witnessed any organized ergonomic assessments in any hospital or office. In a nation known for worker safety and OSHA (Occupational Safety and Health Administration) regulations, the aches and pains are treated as trivial matters. A few hospitals hire industrial experts who are happy to help but the employees often do not know that they exist. In the era of EMR, having a comfortable, productive work environment is critical. Yet this remains a neglected area of clinic operations.

Physician Debt

Medical school applicants are among the best and brightest. They undergo rigorous training for many years. After four years of college, four in medical school and anywhere from 3-10 more years for residency or fellowships, they step out on their own with student loan debts ranging from $175,000 to $250,000 and upwards. This is on top of undergraduate college debt and loans due to other preparatory coursework. Some experts minimize this burden stating that doctors can pay it off quickly. The facts suggest otherwise. Doctors work 80 hours a week during internship and residency and are not paid well even in very expensive cities such as New York where an intern might make $60,000 while still accumulating interest on student debt. Rent consumes much of that. I do not know of any profession which has such grueling schedules and low hourly wages.

Aspirations such as marriage or a dream of buying a home and raising a family are postponed. Recognizing this burden, some medical schools (Weill Cornell Medicine in NYC; New York University; the University of Houston College of Medicine; Kaiser Permanente School of Medicine in Pasadena) are offering free tuition to all students without any strings attached. The University of Arizona in Tucson and Phoenix also offers free tuition to those who agree to serve in a federally designated underserved community for at least two years. Medical and nursing students at Ochsner are offered free tuition for a five years' service commitment. This is a huge step in the right direction.

Debts and Career Choices

Students with high debts tend to choose high-paying procedural and surgical specialties which allow them to pay off debt earlier than those who do the labor-intensive and long-term primary care work in internal medicine, family practice, general medicine and pediatrics. Most physicians are paid well but the so called eROAD specialties (Emergency Medicine, Radiology, Ophthalmology, Anesthesiology and Dermatology) pay far more. These specialties also allow control over one's lifestyle and work hours. Except for dermatology and perhaps ophthalmology, doctors have no longitudinal commitment to patients. Once and done! For primary care clinicians, it is "once in, always in."

Another consequence of the need to pay off debts earlier is the siphoning of great talent from primary care specialties since some of the most coveted specialties are also filled by some of the best and brightest.

According to a survey by Merritt Hawkins, a physician staffing firm, surgeons and subspecialty internists who do procedures bring in revenue for the hospital approaching 5-10 times their salary.[91] Primary physicians are paid half as much because they generate less money and are therefore "less valuable" even though they order most of the lucrative tests and procedures.

The 2018-2019 salary data, based on a survey of 70,000 MDs, shows neurosurgeons earn $616,823; thoracic surgeons $584,287; orthopedists $526,385; radiation oncologists $486,089; vascular surgeons $484,740; dermatologists $455,255; cardiologists $453,515; plastic surgeons $433,060; gastroenterologists $431,767 and radiologists $428,572.[92] Primary care specialties such as internal medicine physicians rarely earn more than $250,000 for laborious hours of "grunt" work. As the salary gap widens, fewer clinicians choose primary care. The income gap is much smaller in Germany and Sweden and their health systems are rated higher than ours.

The devaluation occurs even at social gatherings when the heart surgeon or neurosurgeon becomes the center of attention and the poor internist, green with envy, sips his drink alone! And in a review of over 5000 physicians ticketed for speeding in Florida, tickets were given to 12% of internists/family practitioners and to just 7% of surgical specialists. This was not statistically significant, but a primary care provider might be forgiven for his/her paranoia. Of interest, cardiologists drove luxury cars more often than any other specialist.[93]

Obstacles to Primary Care Practice

Just 6% of our health dollar is spent on primary care. America values and rewards acute care and crisis management at the expense of primary and preventive care. In this upside-down model, invasive procedures are highly valued. This is one of the major drivers of the high costs of health care and a disincentive for physicians to enter primary care careers.

Opening a new private primary care practice is very expensive and it is difficult to find doctors who are willing to join small practices. Efforts to attract more medical students to choose primary care have failed. The shortage affects access, life expectancy and the health of disadvantaged populations.

Even free charity clinics are finding the administrative tasks and EMR maintenance too onerous and complicated. A volunteer-staffed free clinic for uninsured and homeless patients, which was run by Dr. Lynn-Beth Satterly and sponsored by a church in Syracuse, closed on November 19, 2019. Two similar clinics in the area remain open for now.[94]

The COVID-19 pandemic has caused a huge disruption in primary care practices. The revenue loss due to the stay-in-place rules was $15.1 billion nationally or over $67,000 per full time physician. If current Medicare and commercial insurance reimbursement for telehealth were to be withdrawn, the loss would be over $173,000.[95] Small medical offices employ hundreds of thousands of workers in the nation and would have to close if the losses continue. The effect on local economies would be disastrous.

Younger doctors and APNs prefer employment with hospitals or large groups where the schedules are less cruel, the pay and benefits comparable or better, and coverage for time off is easier. They think they can focus more on patient care without worrying about the administrative aspects of a practice.

The cost of hiring a new physician may exceed $500,000-$1,000,000 [96] but the revenue loss, when a partner leaves a practice, can approach $990,000.

Ambulatory Surgical Centers

Surgeons and other specialists, who perform invasive procedures, prefer to stay in their offices or surgery centers. Commutes to the hospital are time-consuming and consultations do not earn as much as surgical procedures. It makes economic sense for them to send their resident, APNs or PAs to do hospital consultations and make follow-up visits. Complex surgical procedures can be done safely, at a lower cost with same day discharges and without the hazards of infections within the hospital environment. This is also attractive to investors and physicians who prefer independence from the hospital's control.

International Medical Graduates on H1-B visas

Physicians who are in the US on a H1-B visa, many of whom care for critically ill patients with COVID-19, fear that if they lose their job or fall ill and die of COVID, they and their families could lose legal status in the US. If they get furloughed or develop a long-term disability, they would have 60 days to find a new job or leave the country.[97]

The US has always been a magnet for immigrants who pine for American educational opportunities and lifestyle - the American Dream. Feared changes in immigration rules are discouraging doctors from coming to the US. The 15,000 IMGs who are here and waiting for permanent residence status for as long as 10 years, are uncertain what will happen to them. They are filling a major void, especially in primary care. Why not just welcome them and get high-quality talent with no further investments needed in their training? IMGs are filling vacant primary care positions not only in internal medicine and family medicine, but also in the internal medicine subspecialties which are generally non-procedural (such as infectious diseases, nephrology and rheumatology). Denial of permanent residency to H1-B visa holders will harm primary care as well as non-surgical specialties.

Overlooked Heroism

On December 30, 2019, Dr. Li Wenliang, a 34-year-old ophthalmologist in Wuhan, China sent a message to fellow doctors in a chat group warning them to wear protective clothing to avoid infection after he saw several patients with what he though was a return of the Severe Acute Respiratory Syndrome (SARS) first identified in the epidemic of 2003. Four days later, the doctor was visited by Chinese police and the Office of Public Security. He was accused of "making false comments" and "severely disturbing the social order," threatened, and forced to admit to his "wrongdoing." He was coerced into signing a letter which he bravely published on Weibo, a web app which allows people to keep up to date with important topics. He became an instant hero. Soon after, he developed symptoms of the coronavirus infection and died on Feb 6, 2020 leaving a young pregnant wife behind.[98] He was simply doing his duty to protect others from what turned out to be the COVID-19 pandemic.

Dr. Roberto Stella, 67, continued to treat patients in Italy even after his supply of protective gear ran out. He died in March 2020, a victim of COVID-19.[99]

There has been an outpouring of support for health care workers during the COVID-19 crisis throughout the world. Clanging pots and pans, singing songs of gratitude and serenading the homes of workers, the public has acknowledged the risks health care workers take to care for the sick. We do not consider ourselves heroes and do not expect adulation. Yet, it feels good to know that there is a thaw in some of the strains between patients and doctors during this crisis. Heath care workers are risking their own lives and those of their loved ones by taking care of COVID-19 patients. For most, it is a badge of honor to care for the sick and scared and some have paid the ultimate price. The goodwill being expressed is genuinely valued by health care workers because physicians have always craved for a partnership with their patients. This could be the beginning of a powerful alliance, a juggernaut that no corporation or politician can oppose.

My profession has flaws which we must fix but most of us work hard and make many sacrifices. We are not all greedy, rude, cold-hearted money grabbers with the big Mercedes and a mansion on a hill. If we have become distant, cautious and fearful, it is because our health care system has killed the joy we felt in the service of others.

Exploitation of Trainees

As an intern in 1971, there were no limits on our work hours. Long shifts, often without sleep, food or water were routine. Self-sacrifice, they said, would make us better doctors. There was no overtime pay, no wellness programs and few pats on the back. We were cheap labor.

Over 50 years, we have watched and tolerated the exploitation of young doctors by a system which abuses highly qualified men and women under the guise of training and toughening. The dehumanizing experience breaks their spirit and sometimes leads to deep depression and suicide.

Physicians-in-training are indispensable for operations of teaching hospitals. Medicare subsidized hospitals to the tune of around $100,000 per resident per year in 2013. The institutional costs are around $134,803 including a salary in the range of $50-80,000. However, the work output of a trainee is estimated to be around $232,726.[100]

In an era when private doctors admitted patients to the hospital, interns and residents did all the "scut" work including drawing blood, starting IV lines, collecting and examining urine and sputum samples, writing notes and calling the primary doctor for orders and instructions. In return, it was assumed the physician would spend time teaching and supervising the trainee by the bedside. The quality of such teaching

SICK AND SCARED

varied widely. I worked at a Chicago hospital for two months as an intern in 1971 but never saw the attending physician, compelling me to look for another job.

Hospitals which employ full time teaching faculty members have more structured teaching programs, but the trainees are on their own much of the time and learn from each other. The time devoted to the teaching of physical examination skills has dwindled substantially over the years. In my own institution, Matthew Burday DO, an internist, has the passion and a legendary reputation for bedside teaching- and several local and national awards recognizing his achievements.

When the work hour restrictions were lifted to "just" 80 hours a week (equal to two full time jobs without overtime), the old guard cried foul. They said the quality of training would suffer. What they were really worried about was the loss of cheap labor, nighttime and weekend coverage, golf time and the decreased time for research or writing. I am not aware of any profession which allows its workers to put in 80 hours each week without overtime. A good consequence of restricted physician trainee work hours was that the hospitals were forced to hire other staff such as phlebotomists (to draw blood for testing) and IV teams to insert, maintain and remove IV catheters, work previously done by the doctors.

Dr. Danielle Ofri wrote a blistering critique of the exploitation of some of the smartest and best trained people one can find. She excoriates health care systems for dehumanizing and humiliating young doctors and describes the adverse impact of long hours on residents and "how they train themselves to accept this self-sacrifice. What other profession in the 21st century would think that 'limiting' residents to a maximum of 80 hours per week could be rational or reasonable?"[101]

Dr. Pamela Wible, who calls the treatment of trainees an abuse of human rights under the Geneva Convention, was featured in the 2018 film "Do No Harm" and is a leading spokesperson on the topic of physician suicide.[5] She has catalogued the suicides of over 1300 physicians. Some have challenged the assertion that physicians kill themselves at a higher rate than other professionals [102] but any death is one too many.

Phillip Zimbardo, a psychiatrist, conducted a social experiment in a Stanford University basement which he had turned into a mock prison. Volunteers, in a simulated exercise enacting prisoners and wardens, assumed vicious roles and behaved as though the exercise was real. At the end of the experiment, several participants could not believe that they had acted the way they did.[103] The experiment sheds light on why some residents, as they gain seniority, may become just as cruel as some of their mentors as described by Dr. Ronald Pies in his essay "Resident from hell." Controlling and shaming others is a learned behavior.[104]

Multiple studies have shown that sleep deprivation causes functional impairment in workers mimicking drunk driving. Nurses who stay awake for 24 hours have risks like someone with a blood alcohol level of roughly 0.10%, which is over the legal limit for driving in all 50 states. Drowsiness leads to a higher incidence of accidents, medication errors and a deadly cycle of deranged sleep patterns. This, in turn, leads to poor eating habits, lack of exercise and health issues.[105] Libby Zion was a young woman in New York whose diagnosis of meningitis was missed and caused her death. The essence of the case was that the intern was sleep deprived. It prompted the rule that no single shift may last more than 24h.

Sexual Harassment and Discrimination

Female health care workers feel disrespected and devalued by patients and peers. A survey of 1719 recipients of career development awardees in Medicine were asked about sexist remarks, inappropriate sexual advances, threats to engage in sexual behavior and coercive advances. Of the 62% who responded, 30% of women reported harassment of some type versus 4% of men.[106] The data is jarring for a profession which has taken an oath of high ethics and compassion. Parity and justice will come with better representation of the sexes in the profession.

SICK AND SCARED

Voices of Young Physicians

An exhausted resident told me a gut-wrenching story about how a nurse reprimanded him for taking a small carton of orange juice from a refrigerator where abundant amounts of snacks and drinks were stored for patients. Now this may seem like a small matter, but he had been up all night in the ICU, with no food or drink for many hours because he missed the cafeteria hours and there weren't any dedicated physician/nurse lounges, refrigerators or vending machines. The institution had no provision for food and drink for residents who worked such long hours. A resident who was saving lives and consoling families was just a common thief in the eyes of that nurse. It reminded me of my own internship and residency days. It should surprise no one that burnout starts early in the careers of physicians. Humiliation, harsh words and other microaggressions add to the misery in a setting where tragedy, pain, suffering and death are daily events.

Older physicians complain that young doctors have "different values" implying that they are lazy, want to be paid well and live well. The younger generation, in my view, is rejecting the expectation of unrewarded servitude to suit their older mentors and the institutions which have exploited their weak position as trainees. Young doctors wish to care for the sick but do not feel self-sacrifice is necessary to achieve that goal. They are not lazy or uncaring. They simply have more commonsense and control than their predecessors did. They are inquiring not only about the hospital and clinic set up, quality, but also about amenities, restaurants, entertainment, and shopping and neighborhood schools. This is forcing hospitals systems such as the Mayo Clinic in Rochester, Minnesota to invest in the communities to attract more workers. Their search for excellent facilities and a good quality of life has been described as the Cheesecake Syndrome which was first described by Atul Gawande who wrote about the restaurant chains' insistence on meticulous attention to detail, excellence, quality control and reasonable prices, all of which are monitored regularly. The restaurant has a huge menu, but they will not serve a steak which is cooked below their own exacting standards.[107]

In comparison, the fee-for-service health care model wishes for, but does not demand, high quality and patient satisfaction.

Changing practice patterns, Hospital Mergers and Acquisitions

Older doctors who ran small solo practices are retiring or dying or being economically forced to accept employment. Younger ones prefer larger group practices many of which are also being swallowed up by hospitals. A salaried hospital job is attractive to younger doctors who do not want the hassles of administrative oversight. These trends lead to greater hospital control over the lives of physicians. Hospital mergers and acquisitions are creating huge behemoths where large systems swallow the little ones.

Atul Gawande, in his essay on the Cheesecake factory, also wrote: "Big chains thrive because they provide goods and services of greater variety, better quality, and lower cost than would otherwise be available. Size is the key. It gives them buying power, lets them centralize common functions, and allows them to adopt and diffuse innovations faster than they could if they were a bunch of small, independent operations."

Apparently, that is not true for hospital mergers which create mammoth health care systems. Beaulieu et al, using Medicare claims and Hospital Compare data from 2007-2016 concluded that such mergers lead to higher prices for patients with private insurance. They are associated with "modestly worse" patient experiences without major changes in readmissions or mortality.[108] Neprash et al reported that mergers do not improve the quality or lower the cost of outpatient care.[109]

Insurance monopolies and brokers

Friends seem to agree with the Nobel Prize winning economist Angus Deaton that physicians are paid too much and are fleecing the system with shady arrangements or outright fraud. Some indeed are.

SICK AND SCARED

But they are not the main culprits. The major insurers (Aetna, UnitedHealth, Humana, Cigna, Anthem, Kaiser, Health Care Service Corp., CVS Health, Centene, Independent Blue Cross and WellCare Health Plans) have a monopoly on healthcare and are reaping astronomic revenues. Their CEOs, some of whom have never saved a life or taken a night call, are compensated handsomely with salaries and perks worth millions. Physician salaries are nowhere close to those of corporate bosses and hospital administrators.

Insurance companies have much to lose if a single payer system with universal care becomes a reality. There would be no need for the middleman anymore. Some companies also orchestrate lies. Wendell Potter, former VP for corporate communications for Cigna, now praises the Canadian system but recalls how employees were told to lie and manipulate listeners. In an NPR interview with Michel Martin on June 27, 2020 he said" amid America's COVID-19 disaster, I must come clean about a lie I spread as a health insurance executive. We spent big money to push the idea that Canada's single payer system was awful, and the US system was much better. It was a lie, and the nation's COVID responses prove it. I'll regret slandering Canada's system for the rest of my life."

Potter continued, "Here is the truth. Our industry PR and lobbying group, AHIP (American Health Insurance Plans), supplied my colleagues and me with cherry-picked data and anecdotes to make people think Canadians wait endlessly for their care. It is a lie. And I will always regret the disservice I did to folks on both sides of the border." He concluded with the executives' motivation for the lying: "They know that if the US moves to a system like that, it would certainly put a real crimp in their profits." He called it a "PR" concoction and "a political ploy."[110]

Pharmacy Benefit Managers (PBMs) earn handsome -and secret- commissions for jacking up the costs of insurance. When costs rise, insurance companies and PBMs raise the premiums, deductibles or reduce coverage keeping their own income and profits untouched.

Some honest brokers, tired of these deceptive practices, are choosing to work for a flat fee.[13]

Preauthorization

Insurance companies hire health care personnel, often nurses, who can veto decisions by highly trained physicians including specialists, based on company manuals. Physicians do not deny that there is some overuse of tests but the phone calls, paperwork and the inflexibility of people with lesser training and experience frustrates them.

Companies claim that they are simply following Choosing Wisely guidelines accepted by most medical societies.[111] But health care is not a rigid science. There is room for clinical judgment, exceptions, compassion and commonsense. An expert's opinion should count for something.

Preauthorization of expensive medicines, while a nuisance, has been mostly a good thing for two reasons. First, it makes physicians think through what they want to do and why. Additionally, it may help prevent the expensive use of medications when equally good generic substitutions can be as effective.

Advanced Practice Nurses (APN) - Pariahs or Partners?

The number of non-physician providers, primarily Advanced Practice Nurses (APN) also known as nurse practitioners (NP) and physician assistants (PA) has increased 441% while the number of primary care physicians decreased 33.5% in recent years. APNs are now the backbone of many health care systems, and thousands more are pouring in. They work in rural America, our inner cities, school health clinics, retail clinics and the VA system, where they were granted full independent privileges in 2016.

Nationally, there is a deep schism between doctors and APNs, each one vying for prominence in health care. Physicians are upset that APNs, who train for fewer years, are equated with doctors who require eleven-to-fifteen years of education after high school to get advanced training. The tussle for parity and respect also has great financial implications because of the salary differences. It is less expensive to hire an APN than it is to hire a doctor, but the salary gap is narrowing.

Some physicians complain that APNs "pretend to be doctors" without the necessary training. But another reason for their reaction is that the APN has emerged as a grave threat to physician careers, especially in primary care. Their numbers are expected to hit 250,000 by 2025. Whether doctors like it or not, advanced practice nurses are here to stay.

Why did APNs leave regular nursing careers? In a Medscape survey, the majority of 10,000 nurses' said that the most rewarding part of their job was taking care of and helping patients; that they were proud of their profession but found several things dissatisfying including administrative burdens, politics, lack of time, nurse-patient ratio and low salaries for the work they do. 85% would choose the same profession and only 6% regretted becoming nurses.[112] What is not reflected in the survey is the fact that many nurses, especially those who work in the ED setting, are burned out. The work is stressful even without the verbal and occasional physical abuse from irate patients and families. Nurses are branching out into other jobs as instructors, quality managers, infection prevention experts, safety staff, risk managers, and APNs etc. Those jobs pay well, and bypass the daily hassle of cleaning beds, wiping vomit, lifting patients, getting yelled at and feeling exhausted and disrespected.

APNs also work in intensive care units and operating rooms as anesthetists. They admit and care for seriously ill patients, deliver babies as midwives, and respond to many urgent calls. APNs help surgeons before, during, and after surgery. They manage chronic, stable diseases such as diabetes and hypertension well and conduct "follow up" hospital visits, all of which saves doctors valuable time.

Many clinics are now manned solely by an APN. Patients often address them as "Doctor" because they too wear white coats and carry a stethoscope. Some correct the patient. Many do not.

Patients are often disappointed to see the APN and not the physician with whom they thought they had signed up, calling it a "bait and switch." Concerned patients should seek clarification ahead of the appointment.

APNs earn less than fully trained physicians, but their annual salaries exceed those of medical residents and fellows who work far longer hours, 60-80 hours a week. Depending on the region, average salaries for APNs are $120,000 to $150,000 and exceed $200,000 for certified nurse anesthetists (CRNA).

Senior doctors seeking an expert opinion in a specialty often get upset when an APN, rather than the specified consultant, performs the initial consultation with minimal or no physician input. As in any profession, there is a wide variation in the knowledge, skills and training of APNs. There are few metrics to compare the quality and safety of APN care vs. physician care. I have supervised a few APNs during elective rotations. In that limited experience, I have encountered APNs who were as good as the interns and residents I taught as well as some who could not perform a simple physical examination.

The number of biopsies done by ANP in dermatologic practices has risen significantly since APN were permitted to do such procedures by Congress to alleviate shortages. Experts claim that as the procedures have risen in number so have lawsuits due to laser injuries. A disproportionate amount is attributed to ANPs. Dermatologists Jalian and Avram state, "…. if providers of varying certifications are performing procedures, they should be held to the same certification, malpractice coverage, and training requirements. Oversight for mid-level providers is lacking. Given the volume of procedures performed, perhaps state medical boards and the American Board of Medical Specialties should have their jurisdictions expanded to oversee mid-level providers providing specialty services."[113]

Hughes et al reported that APNs in general order more imaging studies than physicians.[114] Similarly, Mizrahi et al found that while the national rates for skeletal radiography increased around 5.5 % for radiologists, 11.5 % for non–radiologists overall (10.6 % for orthopedics and 14.4% for chiropractors and podiatry) during the years 2003-2015, the utilization of radiological testing by nurse practitioners and physician assistants rose 441%.[115] Whether this is simply related to the rising numbers of APNs or PA s is unclear.

There are, however, studies which show lower drug costs and better de-escalation to the cheaper oral versus intravenous medications.[116] When complex elderly patients were co-managed by doctors and NPs, there were fewer ER visits and shorter lengths of stay than when there was no NP involved.[117]

APNs now oversee over one billion visits annually. APNs do not want supervision by doctors. Many feel they can do things just as well, and perhaps better than doctors. Sure, they cannot operate on a brain tumor, but neither can general surgeons, cardiologist or pediatricians. With increasing numbers and power, they have become more assertive and feel that they can practice independently. Unrestricted practice is permitted soon after graduation in Alaska, Arizona, Hawaii, Idaho, Iowa, Montana, New Hampshire, New Mexico, North Dakota, Oregon, Rhode Island and Utah. Another 14 states, including Delaware, have a requirement that there must be supervision for some time before independent practice status is granted.[118]

In a new trend, employers are replacing doctors with APNs to lower costs. Fifteen doctors were informed of the termination of their contracts as of April 2020 by the Edward-Elmhurst health system based in Chicago. The plan was to have APNs deal with "lower acuity issues."[119] A Becker's report, which described the APNs in the Chicago system as "mid-level providers," led to a furor from nurse practitioners at Rush University College of Nursing and Rush Health who felt insulted by the label.[120] In 2018, APNs replaced doctors in a chain of clinics in the Dallas area and The Charlotte based Atrium Health System switched its contract to a group (Scope Anesthesia) which hires far more certified registered nurse anesthetists (CRNAs) than doctors.

There is insufficient evidence to determine whether the solo physician, solo APN model or a co-management model is better for the patient in the long run.

Simple coaching and algorithms may make the level of training irrelevant. The show can go on successfully as demonstrated by Dr. Raj Punjabi's work with the Last Mile Health project in Liberia. He was able to achieve excellent public health outcomes by training a sixth grader in resource poor areas to screen for disease and to teach public health and hygiene.[121, 122]

Physicians would do well to utilize (instead of demonize) the capabilities of ANPs' and to also recognize that people who have less training than they do overall, still have a major role in any future reform. Likewise, ANPs' need to respect the broad-based education and experience of physicians and not assume that their education and experience is equivalent.

Physician assistants (PA)

Physician assistants (PA) do not seem to generate as much debate as APNs do. I spoke to Lauren Tavani, who heads a team of physician assistants in the medical intensive care unit at Christiana Care Hospital in Delaware, to understand why she chose to be a PA, what costs she incurred and how she became the extraordinary leader she is. She and her colleagues make rounds, write notes, do invasive procedures and give critical feed back to the doctors. They are confident, poised and prized for their contributions to the team. These teams have helped to reduce our central line infection rates to nearly zero over several years. (A central line is a catheter inserted into the chest or neck to administer fluids and medications for prolonged periods of time)

The PA movement began at Duke University in 1965 where a revered physician, Eugene Stead, saw the need for more clinicians in a time of primary physician shortages. The first four PAs graduated in 1967. The idea gained federal backing and support from the medical community.[123]

There are now more than 119,000 Physician Assistants who graduated from over 200 physician assistant programs. A Bachelor's degree and some health care experience (such as a phlebotomist, radiology tech, Emergency medical technician, and nurse's aide) are typically required for admission to very competitive programs. The first year is didactic and the second requires clinical rotations. They graduate with a master's degree and are as raw as a newly minted medical intern. They learn their skills on the job. Lauren, for example, learned to do procedures under supervision after getting a job in the intensive care unit. Now she teaches others. Senior critical care physicians tell me the PA is indispensable, saving them much time and effort and serving as the eyes and ears for the patients.

The average cost of public tuition for a 27-month physician assistant program was $79,941 for residents of the state and $90,659 for nonresidents in 2019. The typical debt exceeds $100,000. Median salaries for a PA are between $90,000 in Alabama, $102,000 in Delaware and $133,000 in Alaska.[124]

When I retired from a practice with over 40 years of clinical experience, my partners hired three PAs instead of another physician. They are smart, well informed and have been effective. Unlike APNs, PAs are quite content to have supervision although there is a move to have the state board change the language from "supervisory physician" to a "collaborative physician," a term more consistent with the concept of a partnership rather than subservience.

More Middle Managers

Professor Kathleen Sutcliffe, an expert in organizational behavior at Johns Hopkins, notes in her book *Still Not Safe: Patient Safety and the Middle-Managing of American Medicine* that in the 20 years since the publication of the Institute of Medicine report in 1999 about human errors in health care, safety is still a major issue. She blames the continuing situation on clinicians trying to fix what she labels an engineering problem. She recommends hiring more middle managers, psychologists, human factors experts, sociologists and organizational behaviorists. [6, 7]

She writes, "Safety checklists, hand sanitizing stations, posters promoting a safety of culture and programs, inviting low level staff members to speak up" were reasonable "but weak and localized interventions." "Absent were innovations aimed at bigger classes of hazards beyond the scope of even large, multisystem systems such as resolving problems like look-alike, sound-alike drugs…"

We must pay attention to an influential voice like hers. However, most institutions I have worked in since 1990 have had such expertise. Psychologists, businessmen, entrepreneurs, human factor experts, leaders in organizational excellence and doctors with business and/or safety training have been employed or consulted. Institutions saw little improvement, for example, in the number of sharp injuries amongst staff, even after they hired full time, experienced human factor experts. Hand hygiene rates have remained abysmal even with engineering controls and the introduction of extraordinarily expensive electronic gadgets. The number of healthcare related deaths has skyrocketed despite the extraordinary rise in the number of administrators and advisors from 1970- 2009. During this era, costs, waste, inefficiency and harm grew dramatically.[8]

A large hospital hired a world-renowned agency to help with medication errors. I am not sure how much they were paid. Six experts- mostly clinicians who had left clinical practice- met the staff for several days and advised that the hospital hire and train 23 more pharmacy technicians. A previous internal recommendation was that the hospital needed 27 more technicians. It seemed to be an extraordinary waste of money. A senior leader told me that the opinion of someone from another institution sometimes has more weight than an internal one, even if it is identical!

Major sustained achievements in infection control (to be discussed in part 8, The Journey to Zero Harm) occurred only when disciplined strategies such as checklists and "care bundles" were recommended and used by physicians. The threat of penalties imposed by CMS also went a long way, in my opinion, to change the behavior of organizations which, until then, had paid mostly lip service to safety. Business experts did not win those battles.

Disruptive Innovation

The late Clayton Christensen, a business professor and author of the idea of commoditization and disruptive innovation, proposed that physician services can be moved around or replaced without respect to patient relationships. This is the antithesis of the physician-patient relationship.[125, 126] The Harvard Business Review, introducing Christensen's 2009 book titled, *The Innovator's Prescription: A Disruptive Solution for Health Care,* stated: "Our health care system is in critical condition. Each year, fewer Americans can afford it, fewer businesses can provide it, and fewer government programs can promise it for future generations. We need a cure, and we need it now."

An example of disruptive innovation is Netflix which initially started as a mail order business, but it eventually bankrupted Blockbuster's model by streaming movies directly into homes. Health care is already seeing shifts in how care is provided with the advent of retail clinics and urgent centers mostly staffed by APNs. From a business point of view, the traditional physician-patient bond is dispensable if the new system is faster, cheaper, effective for most minor ailments and profitable. But are the alternatives better?

Physicians, high achievers and independent thinkers, do not particularly like others telling them how they should practice their trade. The loss of control over our own destiny has a demoralizing effect.

Devaluation of Physicians

Dr. Mark Lopatin, a rheumatologist in Pennsylvania, writes that systems devalue doctors by equating them with APNs; by demonstrating a lack of trust in the doctor's ability to stay current by requiring costly CME courses; and by demanding preauthorization approvals for tests, studies and prescriptions by someone with much lesser training and knowledge.[127] He describes how Chip Kelly, the famed college coach, was recruited by the Philadelphia Eagles and quickly got rid of seasoned, respected players for younger and cheaper legs. The team did not do well under his command. A couple of years after he was fired, the team was rebuilt and went on to win the Super Bowl.

The message: *organizations should value and honor what they have.*

Loss of Physician Autonomy

Doctors in America were captains of the ship at one time. Current paradigms rightly emphasize teamwork. It is no longer "my patient" but "our patient." Every team member has a right to voice an opinion and to challenge a decision. Physicians still make most clinical care decisions, but they seem to have little influence in making hospital policies or impacting decisions by national medical societies.

Government, insurance companies and hospitals impose burdensome rules which all doctors must follow. They must document everything in a certain format, complete lengthy workers' compensation forms, file appeals, seek pre-approvals, check lab reports, review radiology films, call in prescriptions, return accumulated phone calls, justify admissions, respond to nursing home queries, call consultants, learn thousands of ICD-10-CM (International Classification of Diseases, Tenth Revision, Clinical Modification) codes, ensure accuracy in billing, sign return-to-work notes, complete continuing education (CME) mandates, attend meetings, teach, participate in committees and other duties imposed by the employer, and more. These uncompensated activities, mostly well intended but insidious intrusions, have created havoc in the lives of physicians. The result: for every hour of direct patient care, it now takes two hours to complete other tasks.

The Continuing Medical Education (CME) Scandal

It is obvious that physicians must keep up with the latest developments in Medicine. Learning is a joy when taught properly and without coercion. However, CME, as it exists today, takes much time, costs a lot and has questionable value and is mandatory. Medical societies, boards, states and hospitals demand continuing education certification for continued privileges or licensing. With the proliferation of specialties, many physicians have multiple board certifications and each board requires recertification at regular intervals. One could spend the entire year studying for numerous examinations at exorbitant cost. CME is now a multimillion-dollar business often run by non-physician entrepreneurs for profit.

The typical format for these courses is a conference in a popular city or a glittering resort and even cruise ships. Selected, highly compensated speakers give the same "canned" speech with modifications, year after year. The stiff registration fees, expenses for travel, lodging, meals and loss of income (because of time away from a practice) can add up to thousands of dollars for each meeting. Online courses are expensive too.

I am not aware of any study which demonstrates a correlation between CME, the quality of care and patient outcomes. Many CME questions are esoteric, created by ivory tower gurus, who may see few patients. CME programs have become cash cows to fill the coffers of already wealthy medical organizations. The American Board of Internal Medicine (ABIM) and the American College of Physicians (ACP) have come under intense pressure from members who are begging for meaningful changes in CME. But little has changed.

Reluctance to Unionize

Hospital systems know that physicians are unlikely to take collective action. The idea of self-sacrifice, of giving unconditionally to others, all the time, has kept our profession from activism.[128] That may be changing. I had never heard of the National Union of Residents which represents 17,000 interns, residents and fellows. The Committee of Interns and Residents (CIR), representing this union, recently launched a "Resident Bill of Rights." It asks hospitals, training programs, agencies which supervise such programs and legislators to do the following: give trainees a living wage; act in the best interest of the patient and community by increasing diversity; to restrict work hours to no more than 80 hours a week including non-clinical tasks;

provide time off for being sick without stigma or pressure to return to work earlier; recognize the trainees as fulltime workers with a right to unionize; create fair systems of addressing grievances without retaliation; provide access to mental health services without scrutiny or stigma; fund educational activities; allow representation in hospital leadership roles; and ensure adequate hospital staffing and support.[17]

An effective doctor's union would be feared greatly but physicians are divided about the ethics of walking off the job and have different priorities and agendas. For example, primary care clinicians want to be paid more for the work they do and surgeons, who also work long hours, are not willing to sacrifice their disproportionately higher incomes. Their professional societies have naturally backed what their members want.

As my colleague Dr. Omar Khan points out, "physicians damage themselves through being guilted that they are indispensable, and then complain when no one listens- to our non-existent voice."

Recommendations to Discuss Cost

The high costs of office visits, tests and prescriptions lead to poor clinical outcomes and higher mortality rates. The ACP recently published guidelines to foster cost discussions during every patient encounter. Sloan and Ubel discuss the "7 habits of highly effective cost-of-care conversations." They recommend making these conversations systematic, integrating cost conversation into the workflow and enlisting ancillary staff. They state that "it gets easier and better over time "and refute the argument that costs are "nebulous and unknowable."[129] Other authors reported their experience and suggested best practices.

The CMS requires hospitals to post prices for 300 shoppable services. One local hospital has charges for thousands of surgical procedures, lab tests, room rates and other services. Charges are not the same as true costs and vary enormously from place to place. It is not particularly useful to tell an uninsured patient that a room charge will be $1,705 each night -and more for an intensive care unit- or that the charge for a knee replacement will be $37,000. Most people cannot afford such fees. Physician fees, billed separately, are not included.

What really matters to the patient is what their out of pocket cost will be after insurance pays or, if uninsured, what the total bill might be barring any complications. Hospitals and offices basically charge what they want. The American Hospital Association (AHA) recently challenged a proposed CMS rule that all hospitals must post their charges. A court rejected that contention, but the status of that rule is uncertain. Clearly, the AHA wants to preserve the right of its client hospitals to keep their charges secret.

A recent 15-minute visit to an ophthalmologist was revealing. A scribe took notes as the consummate professional did her work. At the end of an almost perfect visit, I picked up a copy of my record with images of my retina. There was no discussion about costs. Being well insured, I had no worries about affordability. I had no idea what the charges would be and was quite surprised when the statement arrived. Medicare listed the charges as follows: new patient charge $355; diagnostic imaging $145; and "examination with an ophthalmoscope" for each eye was $85. The total bill was $670. Medicare approved $215 and $ 53.85 was covered by my supplemental insurance. So, I know the eye doctor's office was paid $305.68. If I were uninsured, I would probably have had to pay whatever the charge is or skip the examination. Would the eye doctor have known the charges and costs? How would it help? Would I walk out and call all eye doctors in town to compare costs and wait for a new appointment in three months? What is the likelihood that their charges would be much different?

A patient –and friend- recently told me that the system charged her almost $385 for a "complex" office visit, $165 for an EKG, $400 for a chest x-ray, $235 for a 5-minute phone call and $2000 for a probably unnecessary MRI. The patient has an insurance deductible of $4,000. The true cost to the patient is known only to the insurer.

Physicians should certainly be aware of a patient's financial difficulties, but the responsibility for the financial discussions should not be passed on to clinicians. That is a task more suited for accountants.

HIPAA Health Insurance Portability and Accountability Act of 1996 (HIPAA)

An angry patient complained bitterly to our patient relations staff that a physician unwittingly revealed his diagnosis of HIV infection to family members and asked for a meeting and an explanation. Despite a sincere apology in person, the physician was sued and decided to settle. The consolation: the settlement might have been much larger without the apology.

A HIPAA violation occurs when people with no right or need to know hear or read about a patient. Even a wife or husband does not have a right to snoop into the medical records of their spouse without written consent. A conversation with others in an elevator, cafeteria, at a dinner party can leak private information. Records faxed to another office may be hijacked and misused. Hospital employees are known to read patient records of friends or family members without need or authority. Hospitals can be fined for such security lapses. Some hospitals have paid ransom money to hackers to recover stolen records.

Office Bills, Collections and Write Offs

People do not balk at paying $250 to a plumber who clears a drain in 5 minutes (charging you for travel, labor and material) which is $3,000/hour. But if the urologist spends 5 minutes draining a blocked urinary bladder (providing great pain relief and reducing the risk of permanent kidney damage) and charges the same, it is labelled greed.

A patient, who lost his job after he developed a severe spine infection, needed weekly office visits. His wife's two jobs supported them. New to private practice, I asked the staff to waive the $50 co-pay only to discover that it was illegal to forgive co-pay without forgiving the entire bill. So, we, as many other doctors do, completed the treatments without further fees. Bills for hospitalized patients who are unable to pay are often waived completely by private practices and hospitals. I recall taking care of a woman with leukemia for a month fully aware that she would be unable to pay the bills. That cost my practice and my partners a lump of money. Doctors know the hardships their patients undergo and are willing to adjust or forgive such bills to preserve their dignity.

Unlike many other professions, many doctors' offices copy office records and mail or fax them at no charge. We also make numerous phone calls, fill out all multiple forms for a variety of services such as worker's compensation, back-to-work notes, e-mail responses, and we also send reports to employers, etc. for no charge. It always annoys me when some professionals charge me large sums of money for a brief phone call.

Angst in the office

It was another day in the office. I was already falling behind as a couple of patients required more time to address complex issues. I stepped out to apologize to everyone in the waiting room. One patient rescheduled the appointment; another walked out and the third waited to chew me out. He said I was disrespectful for not valuing his time. Unavoidable delays are common. This happens in every office every day. We are stuck between a rock and a hard place. Patients appreciate the extra time taken but those who are waiting may feel otherwise. Irritation turns to anger which is sometimes expressed online.

An essay written by a grateful patient about how her doctors accommodated her urgent needs with an earlier appointment each time she needed it was shared 32,000 times. It was titled "Please, doctor, don't rush on my account."[130]

Clinicians are like assembly line workers; hamsters on a treadmill. Work fast. Maintain quotas. Be productive. Rush, rush, rush. There is never enough time to do everything we must during the visit. We must use our lunch time or take the work home, so we do not fall behind.

Malpractice Litigation and Defensive Medicine

I was sued for the first time in 2014 staining my otherwise "clean record" of 48 years. The patient alleged that several physicians, surgeons, nurses and the hospital were negligent, and proper care might have prevented the "paralysis" of his legs. He did have some weakness of the legs but drove his car without assistive devices.

I reviewed the records repeatedly to understand what I might have done wrong. The sleepless nights, feelings of inadequacy and meetings with lawyers exhausted me. The depositions were oppressive. The details are unimportant now, but I was the first to diagnose his condition, to recommend diagnostic imaging and to begin the correct treatment. I spent at least an hour each day managing this patient and thought I had established a wonderful rapport with the family, keeping the daughters well-informed each day. The events which led to litigation occurred when I was off for the weekend.

I was told the strategy of lawyers is to sue everybody and see who will crack first. Who will throw others to the wolves? Two years later, other doctors, practices and the hospital settled with the family for unknown amounts of money without admitting any guilt. I was now alone. I could have settled too but chose to go to trial because I felt I had done nothing wrong. We hired well known experts to support my consultation. My pride and reputation were at stake. The plaintiffs dropped the case a few days before the trial, but the horror of that experience will remain forever. I had asked my defense lawyers not to mention the patient's self-destructive habits (falling off a ladder while drunk) for my defense. I still had compassion for this patient.

Some physicians have realized that there is money to be made by testifying for or against the plaintiff. These paid consultants are hired by lawyers to review charts remotely. Their opinion is supposed to be based on science and current practice standards of care, but the source of their fees may influence how they testify. It cannot be easy to reject the stance taken by the team hiring and paying them.

SICK AND SCARED

I believe that it is essential for patients to have some recourse when they are harmed. At the very minimum, there must be a timely and sincere apology. Patients whose livelihood is affected have a right to compensation. More difficult is how to place a monetary value on pain and suffering when harm occurs due to human errors.

However, there must be a better way. Innocent doctors should be spared from frivolous lawsuits which result in a substantial loss of self-esteem, cynicism, increased rates of depression, financial stress, callousness towards future patients and even suicide.

According to a Medscape survey of 4,300 US physicians, [131] 85% of general surgeons were sued during their career. The rates for others: urology (84%) otolaryngology (83%) obstetrics (80%), radiology (76%), Emergency department (76%), cardiology (65%), gastroenterology (63%) and anesthesiology (62%). 83% of physicians said the lawsuit was unwarranted. Plaintiffs won only 3% of cases that went to trial. One third of all lawsuits were settled for $10,000-$500,000.00. Insurance companies often urged or demanded a settlement. The main reasons for the litigation were failure to diagnose, complications or poor outcomes.

Malpractice premiums vary by specialty. The annual premium for our relatively low risk infectious disease practice was approximately $15,000 per person annually adding up to $75,000 for the practice. The premiums are higher for obstetricians ($46,000.00 per person) radiology ($21,000 per person) and can be astronomical for surgical fields such as neurosurgery and orthopedics. A few obstetricians I know have simply switched to gynecology which entails much lower risks of litigation.

Fear of being sued is the reason physicians are evasive, wary of patients, order too many tests and practice what is known as "defensive medicine."

The following case illustrates how using clinical judgment can be dangerous. A healthy 22-year-old woman developed a fever and cough during the influenza season. After a thorough examination which showed no evidence for pneumonia, the family doctor sent her home without any further tests or antibiotics. That is a common practice based on good clinical judgment. Most patients do quite well or call back if they are worse. In this case, unfortunately, the patient worsened and died in a hospital three days later. A small pneumonia was now evident on the chest x-ray. The family sued the doctor and won a $3-million-dollar settlement. The lawyer probably kept one third of that. Even if an x-ray had been done, the pneumonia could have been missed in the early stage.

The wary physician orders far more tests than needed to "cover" all bases. It is easy for people to point fingers in hindsight, but clinical judgment, a skill we heavily rely upon, is not always accurate. Diseases can present in subtle ways. The cost of health care is substantially increased by such outpatient spending. Clinical judgment is now a dangerous sport; it's like playing Russian roulette with our careers.

State Laws

Earl Bradley, a now disgraced pediatrician who practiced in southern Delaware, sexually abused numerous children in his office. There were hints and murmurs about his actions, but nothing was done. When he was finally caught and imprisoned, Delaware officials lead by the late Attorney General Beau Biden, whose father was the vice-president then, punished the entire physician community to demonstrate how tough they were on pedophiles. We were required to take a mandatory online course on sexual abuse; threatened with fines or incarceration if we did not report any suspicious behavior; and were forced to stand in line at a police station to provide our fingerprints as a condition of license renewal. I saw no priests, attorneys or politicians in that line.

Legislators in Ohio proposed a law which would find surgeons guilty of "abortion murder" if they did not perform a procedure which most scientists say is not feasible. It would involve situations where a fetus is growing inside a narrow tube called the fallopian tube rather than in the uterus. This ectopic pregnancy can result in a rupture of the tube, hemorrhaging and death of the mother. Urgent surgery saves the mother, but the tiny fetus must be sacrificed. Most experts do not believe, as the legislators claim, that the ectopic fetus can be salvaged by "transplanting" or re-implanting it into the mother's uterus. The legislators in Ohio relied on two reports, one from 1915 and the other from 1990, which claimed this was possible.[132] The proposed penalty for not trying a reimplantation is life in prison or even death. The bill first introduced in May 2019 failed but was reintroduced. If passed, it is certain to face court challenges.

Physician Bashing

Non-physicians blame my profession for high costs, poor service, greed, and lack of empathy. Anne Case and Angus Deaton from Princeton spoke at the American Economic Association's annual meeting on January 4, 2020. Dr. Deaton, the winner of a Nobel Prize for Economics in 2015 was quoted as saying "We have half as many physicians per head as most European countries, yet they get paid two times as much, on average. Physicians are a giant rent-seeking conspiracy that's taking money away from the rest of us, and yet everybody loves physicians. You can't touch them."[133] I was surprised at this virulent generalization from a distinguished scholar. Almost no one else says doctors are the primary cause of the economic crisis in healthcare. Physicians do contribute to high costs with defensive medicine, unethical billing practices, fraud and shady arrangements with industry, but their overall role in rising costs is relatively small.

According to the Commonwealth Fund, there are 2.6 physicians per 1000 people in the US, England and Canada versus 4.0 per 1000 in Denmark, 4.3 in Switzerland and Germany and 4.7 in Norway. I thought supply and demand drives salaries. Deaton did not discuss the relative salaries of other professions in Europe versus those in the USA. Do European economists make as much as he and his colleague make in the US?

Psychological Safety and Peer Review

My friend Dr. Omar Khan wrote "…. our profession does not tolerate 99% right- it seems to demand 100%. If we were wrong 1% of the time (and saw, say, 400 patients a month, which is about right for a PCP) - that means we are wrong 4 times a month and about 50 times a year. Doctors are not given permission to be wrong- our margins are more like 99.99%. Even one minor error a year and we remember it."

Human beings, being human, make mistakes. The lack of time, distractions, overwork, drowsiness, fatigue, depression, lack of safeguards and alerts, poor system designs, sloppy handoffs, short cuts, inefficient workflow, or workplaces without accountability can all lead to errors. Half of all employees state they fear shame, ridicule or punishment if they report their own errors. Hospitals are quick to blame and shame or punish but are far slower when it comes to making real systemic improvements. A punitive culture silences the worker who makes mistakes. Systemic flaws are not uncovered, and the problem continues. It is wrong to punish health care workers, who are highly motivated to care for sick people for errors they commit due to a flawed system of care.

Many hospitals and industries have adopted a system for improvement and accountability called "Just Culture." This standardized peer review system seeks to understand the reasons for errors, consoles workers whose error was due to a systemic flaw, and coaches those who exhibit risky behaviors, such as forgetting to wash their hands or other short cuts, in a collegial manner. Disciplinary actions are taken only when the behavior is egregious, reckless and dangerous. The goal is to encourage reporting without fear, improve performance and promote individual and institutional accountability. The process is standardized using algorithms.[134]

SICK AND SCARED

Is it burnout or moral injury?

> *If you cry because the sun has gone out of your life, your tears will prevent you from seeing the stars*
>
> ~Rabindranath Tagore

The work performed by health care workers is noble and necessary. Strangers in distress seek our counsel and our healing touch. We mend broken bodies, hearts and souls. Our profession has done that for eons. But for the first time in my career, I feel an apocalyptic headwind. The joy of healing others has been sucked out of our lives. Circumstances have forced doctors into a corner from which they see no escape. Burnout is the malady which afflicts half of all health care workers.

The World Health Organization (WHO) refers to burnout as a "syndrome conceptualized as resulting from chronic workplace stress that has not been successfully managed."[135] Exhaustion, negativity, loss of joy and reduced productivity are hallmarks of this condition. Burnout leads to errors, poorer clinical outcomes and lower patient satisfaction. It increases litigation, stress, staff turnover, severe depression, drug and alcohol addiction, and it creates a high risk for physician suicide.

Talbot and Dean argue that it is not burnout, but a "moral injury" akin to post traumatic stress disorder (PTSD). They state, "Physicians are smart, tough, durable, resourceful people. If there was a way to MacGyver themselves out of this situation by working harder, smarter, or differently, they would have done it already."[136]

In a 2019 Survey of 612 physicians, the burnout rates were 79% for primary care physicians and 57% for specialists. Those in the 30-40-year age range were more likely to report burnout. Most did not think their facilities were addressing the issue. Increased staffing, mandatory half days off and reduced patient volume were some of the remedies proposed by physicians. 34% stated they would not recommend their professions to family members stating it is not worth "the sacrifices, financial, emotional, and otherwise."[137] The overall burnout rates for physicians approach 40-50%.

Burnout has existed for decades, but it did not have a name. In the good old days, we were expected to endure the suffering as part of our training, to "suck it up" and "accept the heat or get out of the kitchen."

I read Samuel Shem's (Stephen Bergman) irreverent bestselling book *The House of God* published in 1978, for the second time recently. He coined the term "gomer" (get out of my emergency room) for patients who "never got better and never died.[138] Gomers just kept coming back, deformed and diseased. The non- gomers, usually young patients, had incurable diseases and died miserable deaths. In this state of helplessness, the medical staff resorted to alcohol and drug abuse, sexual orgies, and became depressed, psychotic or manic. One, who just could not cope, jumped off the building, and his body lay splattered in the parking lot below. The doctors were not spiteful. They were exhausted, disillusioned and cynical. Most chose to leave internal medicine to enter specialties which might fit into today's ROAD specialties (radiology, ophthalmology, anesthesiology and dermatology) where patient contact is minimized. Shem became a psychiatrist to escape the ravages of physical illness. Speaking to someone on a couch was far easier than seeing ugly wounds, pus, tumors and death. They had burnout, a term not used then and a condition which was deemed unworthy of addressing.

Medical students start off being more resilient than most other college students. But something happens over time that makes them cynical and angry.[139, 140] The burnout process starts early during internship and residency. Dr. Adam Kay, a British doctor who quit medicine to become a comedy writer and producer of TV shows, became famous for his book "*This is going to hurt.*"[141] He wrote about the institutional cruelty of "inhumane hours imposed on trainee physicians, their often 7-day accessibility and of their sleep-deprived capacity to perform physically arduous and demanding technical work such as surgery for shifts of more than 12 hours at a time."

Dr. Peter Yellowlees, a psychiatrist and the Chief Wellness Officer at the University of California, Davis Health System, asks "Do we suddenly develop burnout because of some bizarre internal development shift that affects only doctors?" He goes on: "Those of us who teach medical students, residents, and junior faculty see the changes over time as many of our brightest and best are transformed from bright- eyed and optimistic to sleep-deprived and skeptical. The answer is quite simple. It is the organizational pressures and stressors, and especially the increased time and pressure at work that we face that have changed us," and "the time allowed for a typical patient consultation has not evolved in tandem with these developments."

"If we are to positively impact physician mental health, resilience will not be the answer. Although resilience techniques can be successfully taught, it is not generally possible to "resilience yourself" out of highly stressful situations. Yoga, mindfulness, and meditation can help, but only so much."

He concludes: "the first change that has to happen is for physicians to learn that it is not necessary to sacrifice themselves on the altar of wildly excessive hours of work. When it comes to burnout and mental health—and to recapturing the enthusiasm of a wide-eyed medical student—the solution is changing the system, stupid."[142]

Nisha Mehta, a radiologist, uses the analogy of bone fractures for burnout. A "stress fracture" she says, is due to abnormal stress on normal bone (burnout) whereas an "insufficiency fracture" is normal stress on abnormal bone as when the osteoporotic grandma falls and breaks a leg.[143]

How is burnout being addressed?

The Triple Aim did not mention the welfare of physicians at all. That came later with seminal papers by Bodenheimer and Sinsky who stated that patient care would suffer if physicians were miserable.[19, 144]

An early study led by Dr. Michael Krasner reported a beneficial effect of mindfulness training to alleviate stress in 70 primary care physicians who were enrolled in an intensive CME course which included mindfulness, meditation, self-awareness exercises, and narratives about meaningful clinical experiences, didactic material, and discussion in Rochester, NY.[145]

The desire to help physicians find meaning and joy in their profession, has led to the appointment of chief wellness officers and the development of wellbeing centers. This is a relatively new concept and its impact is unclear. Many wellbeing centers are led by non-practicing physician leaders, psychologists, managers and statisticians. They teach resilience, mindfulness, meditation, yoga, tai chi, narrative writing and physical fitness. While they do help those who are already wounded, wellbeing centers do little to change the root causes of burnout. Indeed, wellness leaders may not have the pulse of the people they serve or know what truly ails them.

Burnout is caused by defects in a rotten health care system. The nation's burnout experts admit they cannot fix the system. So, they want clinicians to fix themselves, by learning to cope and simply accepting what cannot be changed. Doctors are being asked to cope with something we don't need to cope with, not organize, not demand help. Instead, we are forced into a coping, requesting and a disempowering model. That surely cannot be the way out of this misery. Thought leaders endorse the concept of wellness programs but caution that the goal should be to "mitigate burnout through improvements to physicians' work experience."[146] Dr. Arthur Caplan, a noted ethicist, questions whether the massive investments have been well thought out, planned and budgeted or whether it is just another bandwagon we have jumped on.[147]

Leonard Su, a vascular surgeon who was trained at Yale and the University of Pennsylvania, quit his career because of deep depression. He wrote: "Burnout tends to be treated as an occupational hazard. On the other hand, chronic depression must be kept secret, the suffering to be endured alone." He kept his suicidal depression secret for years. "I've stood on a bridge wanting to jump. I've walked to the top of my hospital's medical tower and only turned around when a nurse called me. I knew if I stayed in medicine, I would eventually kill myself." He continues by explaining that physicians usually "clam up and internalize their suffering. The fear of losing privileges; credentialing and licensing keeps physicians mum about their conditions. Mental illness goes unchecked in those who keep silent. That is what happened to me. Allowing the demon to grow in my mind for years without confronting it gave my worst self-hate a place to flourish".

"I no longer care about how burnout or depression gets classified because I no longer practice. I have no job to lose. I do, however, care about how burnout is treated among its worst sufferers. Regardless of etiology, I know what it feels like to feel that desperate, that hopeless, that alone." And" .... For that subset who is suffering those severe effects of burnout, I guarantee you one thing: all the yoga in the world will not fix their ill."[148]

How do physicians deal with burnout? The results of a survey of 15,000 physicians in 29 specialties to determine how they dealt with burnout were alarming. Negative behaviors included isolation from others (45%), sleeping (40%) eating junk food (33%) drinking alcohol (24%) binge eating (20%) smoking cigarettes (3%) using prescription drugs (2%) and smoking marijuana (1%). Positive behaviors included exercising (45%) talking with family (42%) listening to or playing music (32%).[149]

Testing of older physicians

In 1905, when the life expectancy of Americans was only 50, Sir William Osler wrote about "The uselessness of men above sixty years of age and the incalculable benefit it would be in commercial, in political, and in professional life, if as a matter of course, men stopped work at this age."[150]

It is well known that cognitive function, fine motor skills and physical stamina decline with age. What is less clear is the effect of such decline on clinical performance and outcomes. The data on mortality rates for surgery performed by older physicians compared to that performed by younger surgeons shows mixed results. Older surgeons have higher mortality rates for cardiovascular surgery but lower rates for gastrointestinal procedures compared to their younger colleagues.[151] The mortality rate for patients who receive care from older general internists and hospitalists rises with the age of the physician but that holds true only for those with low volumes of patients.[32]

In January 2016, The American College of Surgeons published a position statement urging surgeons between the ages of 65-70 to consider voluntary cognitive testing. One third of all surgeons are now over the age of 55. The concern was that they might be unaware of, or unwilling to acknowledge, cognitive or physical deficits.[152] The idea has generated much heat but little light. Stanford University backed off from their initial proposal to test at age 70 after a faculty revolt and, in a compromise, decided to test at age 74.5. The University of Pennsylvania plans to test at age 69.5 and Yale will test at age 70.

Late career physicians argue that this recommendation is illegal age discrimination that has no validity unless there are clinical concerns and that it picks on those who are likely to retire soon. The median age for retirement for physicians in the US is 65. Why not test all doctors, they ask, since there surely are young doctors who are incompetent too? What is the proof that such testing improves patient outcomes? We do not even know which one of the many cognitive tests should be used. Who will pay for all this?

Those in favor of testing argue that traditional peer review does not identify impaired doctors. In a study at Yale, where they tested physicians over the age of 70 for reappointment, the authors concluded that "cognitive testing applied by a skilled neuropsychologist is likely an effective approach to identifying individuals with impaired cognitive skills that could affect their ability to practice medicine" and institutions must be prepared to take action to ensure patient safety. A substantial proportion (12.7%) of clinicians aged 70 years or older, some in the 80-90 age range, were found to have impaired cognition, which raised concerns about their clinical abilities and how that "might cause harm."

They stated that conventional peer review had apparently not identified them earlier. They did not correlate such deficits with actual events or harm. It is unclear what type of work the "impaired clinicians" were doing.[153]

My own experience (with what I think is a robust peer review system using Just Culture principles) is that colleagues already know who the impaired individuals are but are reluctant to report them out of misplaced compassion or because they don't want to snitch and fear a lawsuit for defamation. And sometimes no action is taken because of weak leadership at the departmental level.

The US Equal Employment Opportunity Commission (EEOC) filed a suit in February 2020 against Yale New Haven Hospital about their policy to test physicians over age 70. "By subjecting only these older hospital applicants and employees to the policy, the hospital violates the Age Discrimination in Employment Act (ADEA)", the EEOC said. They added ""There are many other non-discriminatory methods already in place to ensure the competence of all of its physicians and other health care providers, regardless of age." Additionally, there were questions about the validity of the cognitive tests they used.[154]

The state of Utah has banned all testing plans after outcries of age discrimination.

The plan to test older clinicians is driving some into an even earlier retirement. What happens to late career physicians? Retiring physicians often simply ride off into the sunset with little recognition of their contributions. No gold watch for them!

The customer is always right

One of the basic tenets of all business is to be nice to the customer. That led me to read Tony Hsieh's book *Delivering Happiness*. He launched Zappos, the shoe and clothing company, later acquired by Amazon. The success of this enterprise was attributed to a happy customer base. The company went beyond expected courtesy and sometimes sent surprise bouquets of flowers to customers or upgraded the product for the same price.[155] It will even manufacture a single shoe for people who have had one leg amputated.

Health care workers chose their profession because they want to serve others. We know our mission. The commercialization of health care, where patients are "customers" or "clients" has made it very difficult for us to do our job. Only 65% of patients now think we are honest and ethical. And in HCAHPS surveys, only 70-80% of patients report good communication with doctors. How can this be?

The erosion of trust and respect has led to patient anger. More patients than ever are abrasive, aggressive, abusive and sometimes violent. They shout cuss words, racial epithets, insult, yell, hit, bite, spit, curse, walk out, throw things, threaten and even pull weapons. Some shoot up drugs brought in by others or smoke cigarettes in hospital bathrooms. Not all such events are reported. We generally just let it go as part of the job especially when the patient is elderly, confused or delirious. We ascribe that to illness.

I decided to keep a tab of reported abuse of health care workers by patients for 30 successive days at one hospital. Female staff members, especially nurses and people of color, were special targets. Sexual innuendo, religious bigotry, racial abuse, threats and acts of violence, were common themes. A highly trained Muslim physician who wears a hijab once told me that she takes a deep breath before entering any patient room, uncertain whether a bigot or racist is assigned to her. Sometimes, she gets thrown out of the room. Institutions often turn a blind eye to the harm caused to workers by such insults, threats and humiliation. Policies to address this, when they do exist, are weak, ineffective and "politically correct."

Patients sometimes reject a black, brown or a turbaned doctor who then steps out of the way to prevent further escalation. The patient prevails and the culture of tolerated prejudice becomes institutionalized. I know several experienced ED nurses who sought transfers to non-clinical positions partly because of the abuse they faced from patients and families on a regular basis.

Critics point out physicians also abuse patients based on race. Clearly, unethical studies such as the Tuskegee study where black men were subjected to experiments to understand the natural history of syphilis even after penicillin became available are examples of abuse. But that was an era when such discrimination, abuse and exclusion was the way of life and often supported by law. Physicians who abuse patients in the modern era should face the full wrath of institutional rules and regulations.

We need a bidirectional flow of kindness to create the bond which alleviates the suffering of both patients and clinicians. Patients must be our priority; but we do not grant them the right to abuse their healers.

Bullying and arrogance by hospitals

Hospitals sometimes mislead, mistreat or bully employees or display double standards. Here are some examples:

Dr. Rebecca Derman, an Obstetrician-Gynecologist, had been treated successfully in the past for alcohol abuse. Years later, a nurse practitioner reported that the physician smelled of alcohol while on duty. This led to a series of events including suspension, a referral to the local Medical Association, an addiction center and a requirement to be tested several times daily for a protracted period. She successfully sued in 2018 for the lack of due process and her peer review rights as well as fraud, defamation and interference with her work. She won a $4.75 million dollar settlement.[156]

Two surgeons, Rainer Gruessner and John Renz, sued the State University of New York system for what they alleged was retaliation (loss of titles) when they voiced patient safety concerns about their cardiothoracic and organ transplant programs, alleging improper medication levels and "a lack of actual patient care."[157]

On April 3, 2020, a Denver health center placed a hiring freeze and asked front line workers to take unpaid leave or cut their salaries due to the COVID-19 crisis. One week later, the executives who made the cuts, granted themselves performance bonuses ranging from

$29,000-$230,000. Robin Wittenstein, the Chief Executive Officer (CEO) got the maximum and Connie Price, the Chief Medical officer (CMO) received $95,792.00. Outraged members of the Denver City council blocked a vote to give the medical center $19 million in Federal Emergency Management Agency (FEMA) money which they were slated to receive. The CEO apologized. But the apology was not for the decisions she made, but for the "unfortunate timing" of the bonuses! [158]

Three Texas health systems ended a 14-year long lawsuit filed by three nurses which claimed the employers, in violation of the Sherman Act, colluded to depress salaries of registered nurses in several cities throughout the US at a time when they were in high demand due to shortages.[159]

Bandwagons and Buzz Words

Americans are an impatient and restless lot. We embrace and discard fads, flavors and fashions as quickly as we fall in and out of love with a shiny new toy. The next bandwagon awaits and promises speed and success. Adherents of revolutionary ideas about diet, exercise, social intercourse, politically incorrect phrases and an assortment of other causes board the wagon and then jump off. Such is the case with health care facilities which spend tons on slogans, statements, logos, rallies and inspirational messages. They bring in "experts," many of whom are not health care workers, to tell us how, when and what to say to patients. Play-acting sessions and videos are used so we can unlearn what we were taught before.

They forget that doctors have been doing this for millennia. Our health systems do not encourage individuality or the expression of unique, if different, views. It is eerie and almost comic to hear employees mechanically repeat phrases which they have been indoctrinated with. They are trying to convince others they are on board, are team members, but sound so phony. Adherence to the party line, damages the unique personality of workers, making robots out of them all. Age-old customs and behaviors are changed overnight as though everything from the past was rotten. In creating new cultures overnight, we lose the collective wisdom (and sometimes follies) of the past.

Sam Rayburn, the 43rd Speaker of the United States House of Representatives, said *"A jackass can kick the barn down, but it takes a carpenter to build one."*[160]

Political Paralysis

Politicians and diapers should be changed regularly; and for the same reasons

~Mark Twain

Americans are frustrated that Congress has done so little to improve our health. Could we not standardize, shorten and simplify all insurance forms, charges, costs and bills? Why can't Medicare negotiate prices with pharmaceutical companies and manufacturers just as the VA does? Why can't we provide universal care for all citizens and have a single payer system like so many other nations which have better health care than we do?

Lisa Rosenbaum quotes Ashish Jha, a well-known health care expert, as follows: "Jha, who is often asked why the United States can't have a single-payer system like those in some other high-income countries, explains that there is almost no health care system that can be transplanted without the host rejecting it. He paraphrases the late health economist Uwe Reinhardt who, when asked about praise for the Danish health care system, would say something like this: Denmark has a great health care system. But if you want me to adopt the Danish health care system, you must also give me the Danish political system, and it would surely help if you also gave me the Danish people."[161]

Opponents of a single-payer universal health care system argue that it would force them to accept inefficient and costly government programs and take away their ability to choose their doctor. They despise the prospect of "socialized medicine" without really understanding what it means. We should be looking at our national interest, not the profit margins of corporations. We should be willing to pay more, so our people suffer less. We should be able to sacrifice a little, in order to serve many.

President Trump, in condemning the "Medicare for All" proposal in his 2020 State of the Union message stated, "To those watching at home tonight, I want you to know: we will never let socialism destroy American healthcare." The plan would "subsidize free care for anyone in the world who unlawfully crosses our borders," and "these proposals would raid the Medicare benefits our seniors depend on, while acting as a powerful lure for illegal immigration" and "…there are those who want to take away your healthcare, take away your doctor, and abolish private insurance entirely."

The President accuses all who think of reform as rabid socialists out to destroy the nation. As Atul Gawande says, "Better is possible. It does not take genius. It takes diligence. It takes moral clarity. It takes ingenuity. And above all, it takes a willingness to try."[162]

The American College of Physicians (ACP), an organization which represents 165,000 internists and specialists, was silent far too long but now has endorsed the idea of "universal health care and either a single payer system or a publicly financed coverage option to be offered along with regulated private insurance."[163] The ACP is the latest of 16 organizations to endorse the bill introduced by Rep John Conyers, Jr (H.R.676-Expanded and Improved Medicare for All Act).[164] As a member of the ACP since 1974, it makes me proud that my organization now represents the views of many physicians. Dr. Tabassum Salaam, now Vice President for Education in the ACP, told me earlier this year that it was a bold and calculated decision by the ACP to enter the political arena.

It should be mentioned the American Association of Family Practitioners led the charge for reform from the outset. It was founded on the principles of equity. It is the largest primary care society, the first one to advocate for health care for the uninsured (1989) and the first one to call for universal health coverage (1992)[165]

SICK AND SCARED

The sixteen medical groups which support "Medicare for all" include The American Association of Community Psychiatrists, American College of Physicians, Medical Students Section of the AMA, American Medical Student Association, American Medical Women's Association, American Nurses Association, American Public Health Association, California Nurses Association/National Nurses United, Falls City Medical society in Kentucky, Health Care for the Homeless, Kentucky Psychiatric Medical Association, Latino Medical Student Association, National Association of Social Workers, National Health Care for the Homeless Council, National Medical Association and the Puerto Rican College of Physicians and Surgeons.[166]

Who are the opponents? A coalition of 115 groups -insurers, hospitals, drug companies and physicians- oppose the expansion of Medicare benefits for all. The ads during the Democratic debates were paid for by the Partnership for America's Health Care Future, a group formed in 2018. Its sole goal was to block Medicare for All, Medicare Buy-In, and public option plans.

The AMA which represents 200,000 doctors (20% of the total) was a founding member of the Partnership. Young physicians and medical student members of the AMA were troubled by what they called a partnership with a "dark money" lobbying group and launched a protest. Lindmark et al write: "After mounting pressure—and just 2 months after the summer protests at the Annual AMA meeting—the AMA did the right thing: It quit the Partnership. Doctors, we hoped, would play an honest and constructive role in the next wave of health reform debates."

Lindmark and colleagues continue: "Unfortunately, the AMA was not the only physician group in the Partnership. Other members listed on the group's website include the American College of Radiology (ACR), the American Association of Neurological Surgeons, the Congress of Neurological Surgeons, and the Virginia Orthopedic Society. We believe that these organizations should follow the AMA and exit the Partnership, and all doctors' groups should avoid such deceptive efforts in the future."[167]

Victor Fuchs, a health economist and professor Emeritus at Stanford University, writes that a single payment system might provide universal coverage and improve health outcomes due to better access. Acceptance of subsidies and mandates as required under the Affordable Care Act (ACA) might also achieve the same.[168]

Crooks within our profession

Medicare covers 56 million Americans. Not surprisingly, crooks defraud the government of billions of dollars thus raising our taxes and premiums. The Medicare and Medicaid Strike Force, operational since 2007, charged over 4200 defendants and recovered billions from fraudulent activity. And this may be just the tip of the iceberg.[169] Sadly, doctors are involved in many of these plots. **Appendix C** provides several specific examples of how people defraud Medicare.

PART 4

HOW OUTPATIENT CARE IS CHANGING

The practice of medicine is an art, not a trade; a calling, not a business; a calling in which your heart will be exercised equally with your head.

~*William Osler*

Outpatient care models are changing dramatically. The COVID-19 pandemic has accelerated the transformation. In a response to the pandemic, hospitals stopped elective surgery, and made efforts to import and conserve personal protective equipment. Medical and dental offices shut their doors. Employees were furloughed. The pandemic changed the face of outpatient care within just a few months.

Practices, on the verge of bankruptcy, had to improvise. The deployment of telemedicine became the safest way for patients to get care remotely and for practices to recover from massive economic losses. Telemedicine was already being used to reach veterans in remote areas. But it suddenly exploded in the private sector as well. CMS and insurers agreed to reimburse practices for telephone calls and video conferences. Emergency rooms and urgent care centers were deserted except for patients who were critically ill. The situation remains dynamic with the possibility that influenza and COVID-19 might create a disastrous double whammy this winter.

No one really knows how this scenario will play out. Some of the changes, such as the widespread use of telemedicine, are here to stay, and Seema Verma, who heads the CMS, agrees stating, "the genie is already out of the bag." As the COVID crisis abates, we will likely see a hybrid model which integrates the old and the new. The information which follows is mostly relevant to the pre-COVID era.

The Emergency Room (ED) Conundrum

The ED has become the principal portal of entry for sick patients who need hospitalization. In the "good old days" primary care physicians (PCP) arranged a "direct admission" with the hospital and continued to visit patients until discharge. That model has collapsed. A PCP will now ask you to go to the ED for assessment and possible admission. Patients without a PCP will also go to the ED or urgent care center because they have no other choice.

Long delays occur when people with trivial illnesses show up. The mix of critically ill and those not so ill creates a problem for triage staff. Creature comforts take a back seat. The glass of water or the blanket requested hours ago may never arrive. A physician will do a quick interview and examination, order tests and x-rays and leave to see other patients or are waiting for reports of tests. The family is left wondering what is next. Patients say, "no one tells you anything." Specialists who were consulted may come hours later -or never- unless it is an emergency. The ED doctor can invoke a labor law called the Emergency Medical Treatment & Labor Act (EMTALA) and demand a physician or surgeon show up. Hospitals may be fined if patients are turned away or if a consultant refused to come in.

Believe it or not, a broken rib or leg may seem like an earth-shaking event to you but is not an emergency for the surgeon. It is just another broken bone which can be fixed tomorrow. The ED will prioritize patients based on what must be done immediately.

Patients feel rushed or neglected and may get angrier when the bill arrives because ED care is extremely expensive compared to outpatient medicine in an office or urgent care center. Even a sore throat can generate a huge bill. The ED has superb doctors who are trained to save the lives of critically ill patients. They thrive on the adrenalin rush of emergencies. Trivial illness bores and irritates them.

More recently, investors have opened "free-standing emergency rooms." They are full-fledged, fully equipped facilities. The distance from the hospital is the only difference. It may be the best place to go to when time matters, and the nearest hospital is too far way.

Urgent Care Centers: Medical Aid Units (MAU) and Express Clinics

Some years ago, during a meeting of the Board of Directors of a large nonprofit hospital system, I asked if there was any plan to invest in outpatient urgent care units. I heard instant groans and sighs from famous bankers, executives, financiers, university presidents and community leaders. Their vigorous head shakes told me that I had asked a rather stupid question. Wounded, I retreated to my safe corner. Fast forward ten years, I was astonished to learn the same system had purchased several existing private Medical Aid Units (MAUs) and had signed an agreement with a national company to develop and manage multiple other MAUs throughout the state. What changed? The short answer is competition, market forces and a desire to establish a large patient base. MAUs provide easy access, lower costs than the ED, convenient hours, and they can manage most medical ailments and become a pipeline for the hospital.

MAUs are convenient places to get acute care for non-life-threatening conditions such as a cut, burn, sprain, fracture or medical conditions which can be managed in the outpatient setting. They cost less than the ED for similar services.

Ambulatory surgery centers

Surgeons usually admit patients to the hospital for any surgery which requires supervision for a few days. They will sometimes consult a hospitalist to manage day-to-day medical problems and take phone calls from nurses. But for same-day surgery, they may choose an ambulatory surgery center.

These centers are less expensive than hospital operating rooms because of lower facility fees, are efficient, have streamlined operations and can adapt, modify and change quickly, unlike the burdensome bureaucracies of hospitals and government. These competitive pressures are changing the ways in which hospitals plan and perform surgery. The ambulatory care centers are also changing the ways physicians are employed. Surgeons, anesthesiologists, radiologists and pathologists can all be independent contractors in such privately owned centers, free from hospital control.

Concierge Medicine and Direct Primary Care

The Concierge Care model is interesting for its ingenuity. Patients typically pay a monthly fee around $100 to $300. This fee guarantees direct access to the doctor 24/7 by email, phone or text as well as office visits when needed, often the same day. Most concierge doctors bill Insurance, private or government, separately on top of the retainer fee. Currently there are 12,000 doctors in such practices across the US. They typically attract high income families earning between $125,000-250,000 and Baby Boomers.[170] I am not aware of data comparing the quality of concierge practices versus conventional private physician offices.

In the Direct Primary Care model, the monthly fees are $25-85. Typical patients are millennials or from Gen X, and their household income is generally below $100K. There are no limits on the number of visits. In this model, there is no insurance middleman since doctors do not accept or bill insurance thus avoiding the costs and hassle of filing claims, hiring accountants and administrative staff. Payments may be cash only. Patients may buy insurance to cover other medical costs. Direct primary care practices can contract with pharmaceutical companies to prescribe generic drugs at costs as low as $2-3 for a 90-day supply in 28 states. They may also negotiate discounted rates for x-rays, ultrasounds, or specialty consultations.

The fee for both the concierge and direct care model ensures a steady annual income and makes it possible to restrict the total number of patients in the practice, often capped at 500 as compared to the usual load of 3,000 or more for other doctors. The arrangement works well for both sides. Physicians who have chosen that path tell me they now have more time to truly care for their patients. Patients seem to reciprocate that feeling. If they were polled, I am certain that the burnout numbers for concierge doctors would be very low.

Dr. Michael Stillman, an internist in Kentucky, criticizes these practices because they are available only to the wealthy, reduce the pool of primary care physicians, manage far fewer patients, and may cater to the whims of patients who wish to get expensive and unnecessary tests or executive physical exams which have little value.[171] Concierge doctors, aware of this criticism, counter that they would much rather provide excellent care to a few than shoddy "care" to many while maintaining their own sanity, family life and their wellbeing. The approbation of others is immaterial to them.

"Integrative Care" models

Integrative health, complementary medicine, lifestyle medicine and alternative medicine have emerged in recent years as an alternative to conventional allopathic health care as we know it. The terms are confusing, so I reached out to Dr. Mausumee Hussain, a US Internal medicine board certified physician who got her medical degree at a top university in London, UK, and now practices integrative Medicine in Kansas. She wrote "a large proportion of the demographic that seeks out integrative medicine, are those that have been failed by or are disenfranchised by conventional medicine." (Personal communication, email dated August 31st, 2020). Integrative Care is often not reimbursed by insurance. But it attracts self-paying patients who believe in the philosophy of good living, well being and healthier lifestyles.

Duke University defines Integrative Care as a plan which "seeks to integrate the best of Western Medicine with a broader understanding of the nature of illness, healing and wellness…it puts the patient at the center of this care and addresses a full range of physical, emotional, mental, spiritual and environmental influences that affect a person's health." Their goal is to care for the whole person; emphasize the mind body connection; reduce the use of medications and focus on self-healing and healthy lifestyles. Noninvasive interventions are preferred.

Who can argue against clean air, potable water, healthy diets, regular exercise, stress reduction, simplification of life, reduction of material needs, forgiveness, respect, kindness, charity, an open mind and laughter with good friends? These are the virtues the new breed of physicians is teaching. They appeal to people who do not want to pop a pill and would rather skip the scalpel.

Hussain added: "Ayurveda and Traditional Chinese Medicine are truly ancient healing modalities. Massage and aromatherapy may also have been utilized in ancient times but were not recognized as discrete healing modalities. Homeopathy was developed by Samuel Hahnemann in the late 18th century, naturopathy in the late 1880's and Functional Medicine was the most recent addition in the 1970's."

Almost 30% of all patients in the US take supplements not prescribed by doctors. When I was in the VA, our HIV clinic coordinator and I collaborated in study with the University of Pittsburgh to understand how often HIV positive veterans were taking supplemental medications, such as herbals and mega-vitamins, which had not been prescribed to them. We found that 1/3 of our patients were secretly using supplements hoping they would boost their chances of survival and wellbeing. Fear and hope drove their decisions.[172]

Dr. David Donohue, a US board certified internist, is the first Delawarean to certify in "Lifestyle" medicine, something I had never heard of. He wrote "I believe that lifestyle medicine is among the most scientific of all fields. We reject commercial bias in all its forms. When you attend the American College of Lifestyle Medicine conference, you do see corporate sponsors, but the scale is much lower and most of the vendors are selling education. When you attend other medical meetings, you see plush gaudy displays and high-heeled marketing reps, and scant mention of disease reversal through lifestyle change." He adds,

SICK AND SCARED

"Allopathic medicine to me seems asleep at the wheel, faithfully peddling the same old therapies that barely make a difference, systematically ignoring the lifestyle changes that have proven ability to reverse the underlying cause of chronic disease, because it is not what we were trained in." (Personal communication, email dated August 19th, 2020)

Conventional allopathic medicine -which I am familiar with- tends to sneer at the new "feel good, do good" specialties. Not too long ago, we scoffed at acupuncture as non-scientific mystical nonsense which defied the rules of anatomy. Now, it is a well-accepted treatment option for chronic pain. The CMS announced in January 2020 that Medicare will cover acupuncture for patients with low back pain.[173]

Yoga was said to be the mumbo-jumbo of devilish cults from India- an effort by pagan Hindus to subvert and corrupt western culture! It is now in every city and state, and the US has not fallen apart! Hussain writes "yoga has been studied to have salubrious effects, especially in reducing heart diseases via a variety of mechanisms. Aside from strength/resistance and cardiovascular training, the breathing discipline induces greater vagal tone and stress reduction."

Preventive care can be prioritized by doing cost-benefit calculations. For example, we would "need to treat 18 smokers with current best practice smoking cessation treatment in order to prevent one death. The price per intervention would be around $500 using either nicotine replacement therapy or varenicline (Chantix). Thus, it would cost around $9,000 to prevent one death." So says my colleague, Scott Seigel PhD, the Director of Population Health Research and a senior scientist at the Christiana Care Value Institute as well as research Associate Professor, Psychiatry and Human Health at the Sidney Kimmel College at Thomas Jefferson University. (Personal communication, email dated July 29th, 2020). Siegel adds "Other forms of prevention, however, are less effective than we care to admit. And in truth, many of the most effective forms of prevention exist in the public health sector, not medicine......most would agree with that idea—it's hardly controversial. But, in practice, health systems are often incentivized by reimbursement rates and not the impact on population health. The net effect, then, is to produce a smaller improvement in population health than could be otherwise possible if existing resources were allocated differently."

The US spends a paltry 6% of all health care dollars on primary care and prevention. Disease prevention and lifestyle changes, blending ancient wisdom with modern science, are important concepts which seek to replace our current US model, which maintains most of its focus on managing acute illness.

What about laughter as therapy? It costs nothing to manufacture or share. There is no patent on laughter. No one can forbid laughter. Osler wrote: "There is a form of laughter that springs from the heart, heard every day in the merry voice of childhood, the expression of laughter - loving spirit that defies analysis by the philosopher, which has nothing rigid or mechanical in it, and totally without social significance; bubbling spontaneously from the heart of child or man. Without egotism and full of feeling, laughter is the music of life."[150]

Dr. Madan Kataria, who popularized this idea in Mumbai, India in 1995, is the father of modern-day laughter therapy. He surmised that a good laugh for 15-20 minutes a day has great health benefits, both physiological and psychological. The initial attempts to tell jokes, both clean and dirty, were not particularly successful. Then he discovered that laughter is contagious and requires no reason! Onlookers, who see someone laughing for no reason, begin to share the mirth. The laughter becomes uproarious and causes bellyaches. The idea has now gained ground worldwide. Kataria offers certification courses in Bengaluru, India.

One time, when a visiting lecturer was in Delaware to teach us how to laugh, I witnessed the entire audience of 100 laughing, tears streaming down their cheeks, dancing, holding hands and running around in circles looking like total idiots. It was a time to be silly, free and happy, if just for one hour. The message was not lost on us. When we laugh, even for no reason, we unleash an inner spirit and joyful hormones notably oxytocin. We give stress an exit path. One who can laugh spontaneously and often is less likely to be depressed, stressed out or suicidal.

Some physicians, exhausted by the pressures of conventional medicine, offer services which we do not normally associate with health care but with cosmetics. Plastic surgeons might do just nose jobs, Botox injections or "Brazilian butts." Some offices resemble spas or beauty parlors, sell mega-vitamins, restore hair with plasma products and hold meditation, yoga and massage sessions. The ambience with beautiful décor, soft music, the strumming of the sitar, water fountains, fragrance of flowers and incense, warm healing colors and inspirational messages are designed to soothe and make their customers feel and look good. These services are not covered by insurance plans. The offices are often owned and run by doctors who have tired of the hassles of American medicine.

It can be daunting to have so many choices. There is a lack of standardization in this world of non-conventional medicine, making comparisons impossible. Randomized trials to compare the models are unlikely to get funded and would have to last years. Hussain feels "the individual patient is the best judge of what works for him/her. Conventional medicine will continue to view it as trial and error medicine, but the proliferation of these specialties suggests that patients are benefiting."

Unfortunately, there are also those who suffer losses to their time, wallet and sometimes health due to the greed or ignorance of unscrupulous or uninformed clinicians practicing what they call integrative medicine.

Centers of Excellence and Corporate Clinics

Businesses are very concerned about the rising costs of employer-based insurance premiums, which are growing two-fold compared to wages and currently average $20,567 annually per employee. They also believe the care their employees receive is uneven. The initiatives launched by Amazon, Walmart, CVS and others will change the way employees get care in the future. Their new designs threaten the current system and are examples of Christensen's Disruptive Innovation.

Initiatives at Amazon

On Jan. 30, 2018, the triad of Amazon, Berkshire Hathaway and JPMorgan Chase joined forces to develop a new model. Warren Buffett is quoted as saying "The ballooning costs of healthcare acts as a hungry tapeworm on the American economy." He added, "Our group does not come to this problem with answers. But we also do not accept it as inevitable. Rather, we share the belief that putting our collective resources behind the country's best talent can, in time, check the rise in health costs while currently enhancing patient satisfaction and outcomes." Dr. Atul Gawande, the well-known author, scholar and surgeon at Harvard, was chosen to lead this effort. (He has recently assumed another role within the triad).

Amazon launched Haven Healthcare; Amazon Transcribe Medical, a voice transcription service with direct entry into the EMR; Amazon Pharmacy acquired Pill Pack in 2018 and partnered with Giant Eagle to fill active prescriptions; and an Alexa enabled device, now HIPAA compliant, can do medication management. Amazon acquired Health Navigator, a startup, to provide technology and services to digital companies and teamed up with Cerner to try to reduce physician burdens. Amazon also selected the Duarte City of Hope Cancer Center in California to care for its employees with cancer. An Amazon Care In app for Telemedicine enables initial screening. Haven is testing its plan in Ohio and Arizona with the goal of providing care to over one million employees.[174]

The Walmart Initiative

Lisa Woods, Senior Director of US Heath Care at Walmart, partners with top health systems that have a proven record of high-quality care and outcomes for specific illnesses. For example, she chose the Mayo Clinic as a Center for Excellence for cancer. Astonishingly, 10% of employees diagnosed to have cancer locally, and approved to travel to the Mayo Clinic, did not have cancer. Walmart also launched centers of excellence for breast, lung and colorectal cancer in 2015 including the Cleveland Clinic, Geisinger, Johns Hopkins and others to get the "right diagnosis and right treatment at the best health systems with the best doctors for Walmart associates." It will pay the full cost including travel for certain procedures. Kidney transplants will be added to the list of procedures covered by its Centers for Excellence program this year. This program is available to 1.1 million people.

The company established a free-standing clinic in Dallas, Georgia in 2019 where a medical checkup costs $30, teeth cleaning $25, mental health counseling is $1 per minute and primary care, urgent care, labs, X-rays, and optometry are offered at prices lower than elsewhere. They want to eliminate the "administrative baloney" and lower their costs by 40%. All prices are listed on digital boards in the waiting room. Patients may schedule appointments and see prices online. No insurance is required. More clinics will open in Georgia, Oklahoma and then nationwide. Initial data suggests that they have already exceeded their volume expectations in their first two clinics. Walmart's clinics are staffed by doctors and offer more ongoing services and a wider array of options than CVS and are in areas where the underserved, uninsured and underinsured live. Their concierge service will help employees find a clinician, coordinate transportation, and find childcare during appointments and address issues with healthcare billing.

Pilot telehealth services for employees in Colorado, Minnesota and Wisconsin started in 2020. The copay will be $4 for a video chat with a virtual primary care physician. Walmart has 150 million customers and their model threatens to disrupt and ruin conventional offices, clinics and hospitals which do not step up to compete.

The CVS initiative

CVS recently acquired Aetna insurance. Their Minute Clinics will expand to include telehealth. After a questionnaire is completed, a board-certified physician will conduct a virtual visit. The cost is $59 and is available in 40 states. CVS plans to open 1,500 new clinics, Health Hubs, by 2021 and the COVID crisis has not slowed those plans. APNs will staff CVS clinics which will serve the Aetna customer base.

Walgreens Boot Alliance

Walgreens Boot Alliance has recently invested heavily in VillageMD to offer primary care and telehealth services across the US. The 300 to 500 offices will be within Walgreen's stores and staffed by over 3,600 physicians recruited by VillageMD. The Houston area clinics are reporting high levels of satisfaction with the services. Online services will be available through the Walgreen's virtual platform.

Pacific Business Group

A San Francisco-based group of private employers and public agencies (Pacific Business Group on Health), created the Employers Centers of Excellence Network in 2013. It chooses physicians and health systems they think will satisfy the goals of high quality, lower cost and patient satisfaction -The Triple Aim. Employers may choose to join this network and by 2019, almost 88% had done so.

***

As the lives of primary doctors deteriorate, does working for these corporate entities generate professional pride? One physician does not think so. The care, the author writes, is episodic, impersonal and its focus is on the current ailment only, too narrow for long term benefits and relationships.[175]

So, while physicians bemoan the takeover of practices by hospitals, these retail industry behemoths threaten to upset the entire foundation of health care as we know it. There is great uncertainty about the ultimate costs and quality of care in the retail clinic model.

The downside of the corporate clinic structure is that these *employment-based benefits would cease immediately upon termination from the job*. Millions of Americans have lost not only their jobs, but also their health coverage, during the current COVID-19 pandemic. Additionally, corporate models may fill a void in health care for episodic care but are unlikely to create a uniform, just system which has lasting health benefits and they do not address how the uninsured, the unemployed and the poor will be cared for.

PART 5

THE REVOLUTION IN INPATIENT CARE

Inpatient care has evolved dramatically in the past 20 years. Primary care physicians found it very difficult to manage an outpatient practice and to respond to the urgent needs of hospitalized patients in a timely manner. That problem was solved by the introduction of physicians who practice only in the hospital (hospitalists).

Hospitalists: From Zero to 50,000

Dr. Robert Wachter, the physician who coined the term "hospitalist," is a senior executive at the University of California, San Francisco. His idea, to create a new category of doctors who work exclusively in the hospital to "cover" the patients of other doctors, was embraced quickly by most hospitals. Whereas there were zero hospitalists in the country 20 years ago, now there are more than 50,000.[176] A typical hospitalist's salary ranges between $250,000-$300,000 and is higher than that of the average internal medicine physician in all states in the US. [177]

Three decades ago, most internal medicine graduates practiced primary care; now only one out of 15 does. Of the other 14, half go into a subspecialty fellowship, the other half to hospitalist work- and of those, some bide their time while applying for a fellowship leading to a lucrative subspecialty

Hospitalists work in shifts. They do not have any long-term commitment to patients. Much sought after and highly paid because of market demand, they vary greatly in experience and quality. Many are just out of residency training programs. Minimum qualifications are the completion of a residency in internal medicine or family medicine, but there is a recent trend to hire large numbers of APNs who practice independently within the hospitalist group. Some work a week on and a week off.

Surgical specialists may also use hospitalists to admit and manage their patients with serious complex issues. The surgeon simply operates and leaves most aspects of the day to day care, including taking phone calls from nurses, to the hospitalist who may complain that surgeons "dump" their patients on them to do the "busy" work.

There are no clear national standards or guidelines for what the daily patient load per hospitalist should be. I asked Dr. Wachter that question when he visited our campus a few years ago, but he was uncertain and noncommittal, because we do not have good data. Some experts recommend a ratio of 18 or fewer patients per hospitalist per shift. Practices, especially those owned privately by investors, thrive on high volume to generate revenue. A predictable effect of high volumes is that there is less time to care for each patient; and consequently, quality and safety are jeopardized.

Outcomes -such as 30-day mortality, readmissions, costs, and discharge-to-home- are better when hospitalists work several consecutive days rather than intermittently. That was the conclusion of a study which reviewed data for thousands of patients at over 200 hospitals during a 2-year period. It is likely that care by a single hospitalist on consecutive days reduced the risk of inadequate handoffs and allowed more time to "bond."[178] A system where a patient might see a different doctor every day or every shift should be a warning sign.

A recent trend is to hire specialty hospitalists who might focus on, for example, diabetes, delivery rooms or trauma units. Some hospitals employ "nocturnists" who are hospitalists that work the night shift to cover the patients managed by other physicians during the day.

The hospitalist, a stranger to the patient, may not have readily available information from the primary care physician about laboratory reports, radiological tests, and may not clearly understand the goals of care such as the DNR status. Thus, unfamiliarity may lead to unnecessary testing or treatment.

Intensivists

There was a time when primary care doctors took care of their patients in the office, on the general ward as well as in the intensive care unit. That model is dead and mostly for the right reasons, but at the expense of continuity. Critical care specialists or intensivists are experts who offer the patient the best chance for recovery. Most ICUs are now led by individuals trained to manage life-threatening illnesses. The patient's primary care doctor may make "social visits," but very few do so. The primary physician is rarely involved, informed or consulted.

The ICU team members, including highly skilled physician assistants and nurses, meet daily for rounds, often conducted in the presence of family members. Consultants are brought in as needed. They are meticulous about hand hygiene and the management of IV lines and catheters. They sedate patients for shorter periods of time, try to get them weaned off breathing machines and strive to mobilize them as soon as possible. Bed sores are uncommon in such units. They have a sense of pride and ownership in the care they provide.

Consultants/Specialists

Consultants may be called in for expert advice by another physician. The patient may not be asked if he/she prefers a specific specialist. And even if asked, the preferred consultant may not be on call that day.

There are certain illnesses where the death rates are reduced significantly when a specialist is involved. An example is a patient with an infection of the blood stream due to Staphylococcus aureus or the fungus Candida where an infectious disease doctor's involvement is vital. Patients should insist on such a consultation for these conditions.

An ethical consultant will not "follow" patients daily during the entire admission unless it is medically necessary. Those perfunctory visits simply increase the cost of care and generate revenue for the doctor. The CMS considers such visits unethical and illegal. It is ok for the patient to ask why so many doctors are making daily rounds.

Rapid Response Team (RRT)

If you suffer a crisis during an admission, someone may call the Rapid Response Team (RRT), and highly trained professionals will respond immediately. The resident/nurse leading the RRT will call the family or a friend with legal authority, with updates after resuscitating the patient. An intensivist is available for further advice. The team will transfer the patient to the ICU if necessary. Most patients and family members are not aware that they too can ask the nurse to call the RRT if their concerns are not being addressed.

Hospital Deaths, Medical Futility and Do Not Resuscitate Orders

Death is not extinguishing the light; it is only putting out the lamp because the dawn has come

~Rabindranath Tagore

Almost 7% of all inpatients (700,000 patients) die in American hospitals each year. The good news: the death rate has decreased 8% even as admissions climbed 11%.

I remember a time when physicians used the term "medical futility" to encourage families to allow death with dignity when the disease process was beyond remedy. Over time, as the patient-physician relationships became less personal, there was a subtle shift that patients and families owned that responsibility. Today, many doctors, fearing labels of paternalism, do not try to influence families but simply ask what their wishes are. Readers may remember the days when supporters of death with dignity were accused of conspiring to create "death panels."

Most Americans say they would much rather die peacefully at home with their loved ones when their time comes. But that happens rarely. Americans are rushed by ambulance to die in intensive care units with innumerable tubes hanging out of all their orifices; sedated and paralyzed by chemical agents, the only sound is of alarms and the hiss of oxygen being pumped in and out of the lungs of essentially dead patients. The cruelty of such existence is unbearable. The futile care causes great suffering to the patient and their loved ones and raises Medicare health care costs dramatically in the last six months of life as patients cling on by a thread with no hope of meaningful survival-largely because they are unwilling to make hard choices before they are left with no choice.

Patients often get aggressive care even though they did not want it. In a study of 1,818 patients over a 10-year period at two academic centers, Dr. Lee et al found that 38% of patients who did not want intensive care received it anyway. They had expressed a desire either for "limited interventions" or "comfort care" only.[179]

Timely conversations with the patient and family members can prevent such tragedies. This is where a good trusting relationship can bear fruit. A daughter, seeking guidance about how to make decisions, asked me what I would do about resuscitation orders for my mother if she had widespread cancer, a massive stroke and no chance of a meaningful recovery. I replied: "I would let her go meet her ancestors in peace and with no regrets for that decision." Her mother died peacefully the same night after the family decided to withdraw all care. A heartfelt thank you note from a grateful daughter was my cherished reward for these words.

Some families prolong the agony for financial gain. Debbie Moore-Black, an intensive care nurse, describes such a scenario." The young wife to this nearly dead 92-year-old feigned love but had eyes on the prize. Wearing a full mink coat, silk lined, in 80 degrees weather, she wanted everything done for Preston. You see, although she would get an allowance, her flow of money would end the day he died." His children had no authority to overrule their stepmother.[180]

A 94-year-old blind woman with dementia developed dehydration and pneumonia. I was asked to see her to manage the infection. She was treated for shock in the intensive care unit and required mechanical ventilation. A nephew, the only relative, instructed the medical team to do "all you can" to save her. She lingered on for a month more with tube feedings, a ventilator and antibiotics. Frustrated staff members wished they could let her go with dignity. The nephew never visited. The staff wondered if he was cashing his aunt's social security checks.

The death of a loved one is tragic under any circumstance, but death in a hospital can be even more traumatic. Survivor support systems may be insufficient or nonexistent. Patients often die lonely deaths. This has been a major issue during the current COVID-19 crisis when isolation policies are causing patients to die alone, untouched by loved ones. If a death occurs during off hours, the resident on call who does not know the person will sign a death certificate. The consolation by chaplains they have never met before is valuable, but impersonal.

In a nation where loneliness is estimated to affect 17% of the population, it is not uncommon to meet patients who have no family or friends. They die alone, un-mourned and are sometimes buried in anonymous cemeteries for the indigent. My institution, Christiana Care, launched a program titled "No one dies alone." Volunteer staff members took turns to sit with any patient who wanted company until the very end. These are the heroes in health care few write about.

Does external oversight by a regulatory agency affect death rates? A study, conducted in 1,984 hospitals, assessed the effect of 3,417 unannounced Joint Commission (JC) visits from 2008-2012 on 30-day inpatient mortality rates. Patients admitted during the week of a survey had a significantly lower mortality rate than did patients admitted during the three weeks before. The overall mortality rate went down by 1.5% but by 5.9% for major teaching hospitals. The conclusion: changes in practice occur during survey periods which reduce mortality perhaps due to fewer medical errors.[181]

Does the day and time of the week influence mortality? In a study of 30-day mortality rates for emergency admissions during weekends, holidays and nights in the UK over a 10-year period (2004-2014), within or outside the hospital, Dr. Lu et al found that the mortality was higher than at other times. This effect was additive, so the risk of death was higher on a weekend night. Whether this is due to understaffing, a lower availability of resources or diagnostic facilities or due to the "B-team" being on call at those times is unclear.[182] The implication is that one is safer if hospitalized on weekdays during regular working hours when the staffing is best.

Hospital rules require that patient preferences about cardiopulmonary resuscitation (CPR) be documented. These wishes must be signed by an attending physician. When the patient requests no CPR, an order called "do not resuscitate" (DNR) is placed in the chart and allows natural death. Without the DNR order, health care workers will descend on the bewildered, dying patient, pound on the chests of frail men and women, break their ribs, shock them, poke them with needles and catheters and leave a bloody scene reminiscent of a battlefield. Even a DNR order is no guarantee that things will go as planned. In crisis situations, when time is of the essence, health care workers may inadvertently forget to check for such a designation.

Discharge planning

Discharge from the hospital is a laborious, time-consuming task for doctors and a confusing, hazardous time for patients. Discharges are conducted when convenient for the system rather than to suit the patient and the family. While average hospital stays are 4-5 days, many patients remain in the hospital longer because of poor planning. Insurers may not pay hospitals for the "extra days." Weekend and evening discharges are uncommon in order to suit physician schedules and convenience.

Rapid-fire instructions, replete with medical jargon, are completed in a couple of minutes, followed by "do you understand?" rather than "could you please repeat for me what the instructions are, so I know there is no confusion?" A sheaf of papers is handed over for the obligatory signatures. Patients often nod affirmatively because they don't want someone to think they are slow or stupid. Most of the instructions are forgotten within minutes. I suspect many patients never read the paperwork handed over to them.

Discharge summaries, an essential repository of information, range in quality from superb to worthless. Hospitals do not check the quality of the discharge summary. They are interested only in whether it was completed and signed, so billing may proceed. It is rare for the discharging doctor to call the PCP to hand off the patient, even as a matter of courtesy.

A physician told me that after his appendectomy, nobody gave him discharge instructions and his prescriptions included two medicines – one which had been discontinued months ago and the other one had caused a severe reaction- even though he had specifically asked the team to delete these medications from the list. Caretakers receiving a confused or debilitated patient would follow the instructions on the form.

Transfers to Nursing Home

Discharging to a nursing home is also a dangerous time for patients. The transition is often clumsy and incomplete. Records might not accompany the patient. Hospital physicians do not call nursing home physicians, or nurses, to share information. Nursing homes are known to send patients right back to the hospital because the patient they received was cold, blue and in shock. The dangers of nursing home transfers will be discussed in some depth in Part 8, The Journey to Zero Harm.

Hospital to Hospital Transfers

Most inter-hospital transfers for higher level management are cordial and well-coordinated but receiving physicians may speak in an unprofessional or condescending manner to professionals at smaller hospitals or emergency rooms. There is an ongoing paranoia that smaller hospitals "dump" patients on larger referral centers especially on Fridays and weekends so their own specialists can go to the beach! When transfers do occur, the patient may arrive with no records and/or unable to provide a decent history.

Hospitals with the appropriate resources to treat a patient are not permitted to reject a patient from another institution which lacks that capability. That would be a violation of the labor law called EMTALA.

Medical Tourism and "Travel Surgery" Practice

Medical tourism has become a big business. A few nations in South America and Asia have built ultra-modern hospitals with the latest equipment, staffed by highly trained physicians and surgeons. Their goal is to lure patients from rich nations. Patients are treated like celebrities in these high quality and aesthetically pleasing facilities at a cost much lower than in western nations. Incentives may include all post-op and rehab care, spa-like conditions and a vacation bundled into the package. Indian immigrants from all over the world and many wealthy Arabs go to India for complex medical issues, joint replacements, dental care and cataract surgery. They get great care, a chance to meet relatives and assurance that it will be affordable.[183]

Chuck Selvaggio, the executive director of the Neighbors to Nicaragua Inc. philanthropy, wrote: "...in Nicaragua, many American dentists retire to practice because of the lack of 'red tape' (administrative requirements and insurance) that is omnipresent in the USA. Consequently, many Americans go to Nicaragua for low-cost/high quality dental work." (Personal communication, email dated August 12th, 2020)

The general perception in the US is that overseas facilities have poor hygiene, high infection rates, untrained staff and uneven outcomes. That is indeed true for many foreign -and American- hospitals, but the ones that cater to medical tourists maintain very high standards and invite inspections from certifying bodies such as the Joint Commission. Friends who were posted in India, Germany and China report very high satisfaction with the quality of medical and surgical care when they faced medical emergencies. The physicians and surgeons are often highly experienced, multilingual and trained in western countries.

Some US insurance companies, including Blue Cross and Blue Shield, have packages to fly patients to selected hospitals and will waive some of the costs because they too benefit from the cost savings. However, most insurance policies do not cover services overseas unless it is an emergency. Medicare does not cover health care outside US territories.

James Polsfut, previously an executive at General Electric, is now the CEO of North American Specialty Hospital based in Denver. His company has contracts with US companies comprising 3 million people. Patients, who need joint replacement surgery or costly drug infusions, get pre-op care from US based physicians. The patients and the surgeon then travel to the Galenia Hospital in Cancun, Mexico, for the surgery or infusion and return to the US for post-op care. Remarkably, the surgeons make twice as much for each procedure since the costs of labor and supplies are much lower in Mexico.[184]

PART 6

TECHNOLOGY: SERVANT OR MASTER

Kevin Kelly, the tech guru, wrote:

"This is not a race against the machines. If we race against them, we lose. You'll be paid in the future based on how well you work with robots."

"We need to let robots take over. Many of the jobs that politicians are fighting to keep away from robots are jobs that no one wakes up in the morning really wanting to do. Robots will do jobs we have been doing and do them much better than we can. They will do jobs we can't do at all. They will do jobs we never imagined even needed to be done. And they will help us discover new jobs for ourselves, new tasks that expand who we are. They will let us focus on becoming more human than we were."

"It is inevitable. Let the robots take our jobs and let them help us dream up new work that matters."[185]

Estimates vary but there will be a need for 150,000 to 350,000 more health care workers within two decades.[186] The need will be especially acute for primary care, home health services and long-term care facilities as the population ages and the labor pool shrinks. These are tough jobs which do not pay well. Robots may be able to perform some of the tasks. In an interesting experiment at the Knollwood Military Community in Washington DC, a team from the Innovation lab at Trinity College, Dublin, is using "Stevie," a robot which can sing, help with Bingo, answer 100 questions, has a computer interface, can smile and do a "clumsy dance." It amuses and entertains residents who find it good company.[187]

Robots already deliver medications in hospitals and food in restaurants. Drones will soon drop prescriptions at your doorstep. Properly programmed machines can be smart, accurate, consistent and reliable. They do not get bored or tired; they work 24/7 and do not complain! As Ken Jennings, the Jeopardy champion and several chess masters found out, they are no match for IBM's Watson.

Patients might find gadgets, which are now ubiquitous in American homes, to be an ally in their health care. Amazon recently partnered with a company called ShareCare to incorporate 80,000 health related questions onto the Alexa platform. One can ask Alexa questions such as "when will the flu season start?" or "when should people get a colonoscopy?"

Intelligent machines could gather a good history (a lost art in Medicine) before the physician enters the room and use algorithms to provide clues to a diagnosis. Time constraints have made it so difficult for physicians to take a thorough history and perform a decent physical examination that many are losing these critical skills. There is a joke about the "orthopedic point," (with apologies to my orthopedic friends and colleagues) which is a brief ritual where the surgeon places his stethoscope in the area just above the belly button, hears heart sounds, air moving in and out of lungs and the gurgling of stomach contents; takes a quick look to see if the limbs are moving; whether the skin is intact. He/she then checks one box in a template, indicating that a complete head to toe examination was performed. Orthopedic surgeons, however, are not the only physicians who take such short cuts.

I have seen clinicians listen to the lungs for a few seconds through three layers of thick winter clothing simply to avoid the accusation that "he did not even touch me." These acquired bad habits lead to less confidence in one's own bedside exam skills and the greater use of technology. Nowadays, it is common for physicians to order a CT scan before the physical examination, simply based on the symptoms because it is known that the scan is more accurate in picking up certain diagnosis such as appendicitis or early pneumonia.

Davenport and Kalakota have summarized well what artificial intelligence (AI) may offer to health care.[188] For example, AI can speed up the diagnostic accuracy in conditions such as psychosis, cancer, pigmented skin lesions or genetic diseases.[189]

Eko is a software company which uses AI to analyze heart sounds data gathered by noninvasive sensors. Its algorithm outperformed four out of five cardiologists in detecting pediatric heart murmurs.[190]

A deep learning algorithm identified bleeding in the brain with great accuracy and was better than two of four board certified radiologists who read the same CT scans. It is also faster and could decrease costs and misdiagnosis. Radiologists plus the algorithm might do even better.[191]

Periodic eye examinations can prevent retinal damage and blindness, especially for those with diabetes and hypertension, but only 50% of high-risk patients get regular eye examinations. It is hard to find an ophthalmoscope on hospital units; few doctors carry one and even fewer know how to use the instrument properly. In 2018, the FDA approved a screening tool developed by Idx Technologies (Idx-DR) for diabetic retinopathy after extensive trials over 10 years. The easy to use tool could be deployed in primary care clinics and even grocery stores. A high school student can be trained to use it effectively. Another deep learning system using photographs of the fundus of the eye was able to identify swollen optic disks (papilledema), normal disks and other abnormalities accurately.[192]

BlueDot is a health monitoring platform in Canada which was created in 2014 by Dr. Karam Khan, an infectious disease expert who had experienced the 2003 Severe Acute Respiratory Syndrome (SARS) outbreaks in Toronto firsthand and remembered the chaos. He created an algorithm which predicted the spread of the current coronavirus outbreak on Dec 31, 2019, six days before the CDC and nine days before the WHO. The algorithm uses machine learning, artificial intelligence, animal and plant disease networks, and airline ticketing information to predict the spread of the infections. In the case of COVID-19, they used airline ticketing information to predict the spread of the virus from Wuhan to other countries in Asia.[193]

AI is not perfect. The Stanford Apple Study was a bold experiment to see if an app could identify a dangerous irregular rhythm known as atrial fibrillation. Participants used a smartphone (Apple iPhone) app and gave consent to be monitored. If an irregular pulse was identified, the individual received notification and called a number to initiate a telemedicine visit. An electrocardiography (ECG) patch was mailed to the participant, to be worn for up to seven days. Surveys were administered 90 days after notification of the irregular pulse and at the end of the study. Only 2,161 (0.5%) participants had an irregular rhythm. Atrial fibrillation was confirmed in only 34%, suggesting low sensitivity and specificity in this study to identify this rhythm disturbance.[194] Many participants did not bother to call.

Inadvertent racial bias in algorithms was reported by Ziad Obermeyer et al in a study where they tested a commercially available algorithm - Impact Pro, from Optum- in a large population (6,079 black and 45,539 white) and found that for a given score, black patients were "considerably" sicker, and their illness was uncontrolled. If the bias were removed, 46.5% of black patients would have become eligible for more care compared to 17.7% identified by the algorithm.[195]

Some algorithm-based apps perform poorly in detecting skin cancer, especially with darker skin. This may be due to small sample sizes, poor photographs, and unrepresentative populations. This will need more attention before the technology can be deployed widely.[196, 197]

Geralyn Miller, a director of AI and research at Microsoft, writes: "Perhaps most important, we need diversity, because AI works only when it is inclusive. To create accurate models, we need diversity in the developers who write the algorithms, diversity in the data scientists who build the models and diversity in the underlying data itself." She states that to be truly successful, "we will need to overlook the things that historically set us apart, like race, gender, age, language, culture, socioeconomic status and domain enterprise."[198]

Physicians are not threatened by technology and embrace its value and potential. Even those who scorn the EMR are not willing to revert to paper charts again. Physicians are increasingly relying on technology to confirm their clinical findings. For example, a suspected pneumonia may be confirmed by a chest x-ray which might be more reliable than a physical examination, especially in these times of deteriorating clinical skills. One may ask a gastroenterologist to place a tube in the stomach to confirm that the suspected ulcer is indeed present.

The principle of wanting to do the best we can diagnostically and therapeutically for our patient remains as sound now as it ever was. We will embrace technology to do it. The question is whether we will find a balance between the coldness of the machine and the warmth of a human hand?

Telehealth

The growth of telehealth has accelerated dramatically from 13,000 visits weekly before the COVID-19 crisis to more than 1.7 million and rising now. The VA already had several tele-health programs for primary and specialty care geared towards veterans who live in remote areas. Recently, the VA partnered with Apple to provide 50,000 cellular connected devices (iPads) with special software to eligible veterans who lack internet access.

Medicare and many insurers approved payments for virtual care during the COVID-19 crisis. But while Seema Verma, the CMS administrator admits telehealth is here to stay, some insurers are already balking at the cost. It eats into their profits. The advantages of virtual care are obvious: quick and easy access, no transportation requirements, lower cost, and the ability to do frequent monitoring. It is especially useful for those in rural areas, the frail, and the elderly, the economically-disadvantaged, and the disabled. And hand hygiene may matter less!

As we are learning with school programs using Zoom, online education might become a popular trend for diabetic classes, diet advice, cancer screening, vaccination information, counseling, consoling and simply connecting vulnerable populations to health care.

There is, of course, some trepidation. The University of Michigan in partnership with the American Association of Retired Persons (AARP) surveyed 2,000 people age 50-80 in May 2019 and found that 71% were concerned that a remote physician examination might not be feasible; 68% worried about the quality of care; 49% had concerns about privacy and lack of personal connection; 55% did not know if their own health system offered it. Only 4% had had a televised visit during the past year.[199] A follow-up study was conducted by the same group during the COVID era (March-June 2020). The number of telemedicine encounters had risen from 4% to 26% within months. Confidence in this type of visit increased from 53% to 64%. However, the attitudes about the absence of a physical examination, the quality of care or the lack of a personal connection did not change. Concerns about privacy did go down from 49% to 24%. Twenty five percent of those surveyed were worried about not hearing well or seeing items during a telemedicine visit.

It is now also possible to "examine" patients remotely with sophisticated instruments/cameras in the patient's home. There is no doubt that our capabilities for remote examinations will improve over time.

Teladoc Health announced in October 2019 that they have launched Teladoc Medical Experts "the first-of-its-kind, broad-based virtual center of excellence for individuals dealing with a wide range of complex and/or costly mental and physical medical needs. With this unique service, a state-licensed doctor works directly with individuals, regardless of their geographic location, to get timely answers regarding accurate diagnoses and treatment plans advice." Teladoc Medical Experts is currently available for more than 100,000 members across the U.S. It delivers care in 130 countries and in more than 30 languages. It partners with employers, hospitals and health systems, and insurers to transform care delivery.[200]

Baby boomers — those between age 54-73- only 46% of whom use technology (other than carrying cell phones or using keyboards) — may find the transition a bit more challenging compared to Gen X (age 39-53) or millennials (age 24-38) and Gen Z (age 18-23) who use the technology 65%, 76% and 74% of the time, respectively.[201]

But over 36 million Americans cannot read or write, and many more do not have access to computers and broadband internet. How will they access Telehealth?

PART 7

FIRST, DO NO HARM

Primum non nocere

Total strangers ask us to protect them from disease and death. Physicians become their confidants, the hospital their refuge. Grateful patients send thank you notes for endless acts of kindness. We store the treasured words forever and are inspired to do more. We write powerful, emotional and dramatic essays about how meaningful our interactions with patients are to us; how the suffering of patients is internalized by their doctors who suffer just as much. For anyone who wants to gauge the range of emotions doctors feel, I recommend the book titled *A Piece of My Mind*, a compilation of essays which is guaranteed to move the reader.[202] These are selected essays from thousands which were submitted to the *Journal of the American Medical Association* (JAMA). Particularly poignant are the descriptions of the deaths of the elderly, loved ones, and children.

The words, *primum non nocere* (First, do no harm) are often believed- erroneously- to be a part of the Hippocratic Oath that physicians take when they complete their medical training. The goals of the profession to heal would make such an oath redundant anyway. Intentional harm is extremely rare in health care.

Dr. Derek Feeley, in his introduction of *"A framework for Safe, Reliable and Effective Care,"* wrote that a culture of safety requires learning what went wrong, being proactive, creating better systems, being humble and transparent, working with families and recognizing that safety is not just the absence of physical harm, but also the "pursuit of dignity and equity" in health care.[203]

Despite our best intentions, however, injuries or deaths from preventable errors are common. The fact that much of the care we provide is safe and good does not mitigate the suffering of afflicted patients and families. Each one is a tragedy, an opportunity to improve and to learn from.

My goal is to inform, not alarm. The stories, which are recalled from memory, are just a tiny fraction of all the tragedies within the health care system. Far too often, the learning afforded by these harm events does not translate into real change. A huge opportunity to make health care safer is then lost because of institutional lethargy and the lack of leadership.

Reckless behavior by clinicians, when the risk of causing harm is apparent, must be punished. However, it is unrealistic to expect that they will not make occasional mistakes. Safe hospitals anticipate human frailty and build safeguards to catch the errors in a timely manner. To do otherwise is cruel. I have classified the harm events in four broad categories, but there are *many overlaps* among the groups.

1. Harm due to acts of omission or commission.
2. Harm due to lapses in communication.
3. Harm due to faulty systems within healthcare.
4. Other causes of harm.

1. Harm due to Acts of Omission or Commission

Shock

A young mother's blood pressure dropped to shock levels (66/40 mm/Hg) a few hours after she had major spine surgery. During the night, the nurse first called an APN, then two doctors two hours apart. All of them ordered increasing amount of IV fluids. None of them reviewed the chart, examined the patient or called the nurse back to ask if the patient was stable. The surgeon was completely unaware of these developments. Finally, the exhausted nurse called the Rapid Response Team (RRT) which brought nurses and physicians to the bedside immediately for proper care. The APN said she was overwhelmed with admissions and phone calls, and her back up physician was at another hospital. That is a hospital system issue and the APN cannot be blamed for being forced into an untenable position. The doctors acknowledged that they had failed to respond appropriately when called. The patient survived despite critical omissions in care. The hospital changed the coverage system to get more help for the APN during the night shift. The doctors expressed regret and were coached to make safer choices.

The problem: Not reviewing the records or examining the patient especially after the initial fluid challenge had failed and a faulty system of on call coverage.

A Fatal Hospital Acquired Infection

Ms. Carole Hemmelgarn is a well-known safety expert who lost her nine-year-old daughter Alyssa ten days after a diagnosis of acute lymphocytic leukemia, a highly curable condition in children. The cause of death was a severe bowel infection due to Clostridioides difficile (C. diff) bacteria and sepsis after just 2-3 courses of chemotherapy.

There was initial silence, lack of disclosure and mounting frustration. Carole, with experience in the health care industry, felt a deep range of emotions - guilt, shame, sadness and despair –which persist today. (Personal Communication, email dated July 23, 2020).

The tragedy led to her getting her two master's degrees in Patient Safety and Leadership as well as Health Care Ethics. She is now an adjunct Professor at the University of Illinois, Chicago and Georgetown University in Washington D.C. and serves as a board member on the Board Quality, Safety & Experience Committee at the hospital in Denver where Alyssa died. The Alyssa Cares Foundation honors the memory of this beautiful child and distributes books to children.[204]

The problem: Likely a breakdown in hand hygiene and infection prevention measures which permitted this acquisition of this infection in the hospital. The disclosure was delayed and clumsy.

Perforation

An elderly man fell at home and was treated successfully for severe dehydration and kidney failure. A few nights later, he developed new, agonizing abdominal pain with black, tarry stool (which implies bleeding within the intestines or stomach). The nurse inexplicably did not call the MD for hours. The MD, when called, did not examine the patient but told the nurse to give the patient an antacid. The autopsy revealed a perforated stomach ulcer—likely due to the severe stress from illness-with bleeding and infection. A surgeon could have saved the patient. The death occurred in a facility with world-class talent and equipment. Earlier communication by the nurse and a more expeditious approach by the doctor might have prevented the death. Was this simply poor judgment or laziness?

The problem: Not reporting and responding quickly to a major change in the patient's condition. The disclosure was delayed and inadequate..

A missed mass

A patient with chest discomfort underwent a cardiac catheterization procedure (injecting dye in the blood vessels of the heart) to rule out coronary artery disease. If someone had looked at the chest x-ray, or read the report, or taken a better history, or done a better physical examination, they would have discovered that the cause of the pain was a large lung tumor. He needed a cancer specialist, not a cardiologist. The error was discovered six months later when the tumor had already spread to the brain. The family, following an honest disclosure, forgave the physician who had apologized to the family.

The problem: an incomplete patient evaluation and review of records.

SICK AND SCARED

Tuberculosis (TB)

Two friends paid a heavy price when clinicians failed to treat them for positive blood or skin test results for TB. The tests indicated that they were exposed to TB in the past and the bacteria were still "hiding" (latent) in the body. They should have received treatment for the latent TB infection because they were on medications which damage the immune system and allow the TB to become active. One developed TB of the lungs which almost killed her. The other, treated at an Ivy League medical school for cancer, was cured of the cancer but died of widespread TB. Individuals who are born outside the US, especially in Asia and Africa, should be tested for TB with a simple blood or skin test and treated if they are at risk for activating the hidden bacteria.

The problem: lack of knowledge or dismissal of a major public health issue especially in immigrants.

Wrong patient

A nurse prepared a patient for a pelvic examination. Shortly thereafter, a physician walked in and, without a word, proceeded with the exam. Shortly thereafter, both the physician and patient realized they did not know each other. The doctor had entered the wrong room.

The problem: Not only did he not confirm the identity but also bypassed common courtesy in doing a very private and sensitive examination.

A swollen neck

A central IV line (a thin tube placed in a vein to provide intravenous fluids and medications) was inserted successfully in the neck, but after a few hours, a nurse noted swelling and discoloration around the insertion site. The swelling was noted to be somewhat larger after four hours. The patient should have been monitored closely for bleeding but was left unmonitored for the night and found dead the next morning. He had a massive internal hemorrhage. This was a preventable death. A full disclosure was made to the family.

The problem: Inadequate monitoring of an enlarging life-threatening hematoma after a procedure.

Brain Damage

A 49-year-old man mistakenly received an antibiotic before a surgical procedure even though he had a well-documented, life-threatening allergy to it. Soon after receiving the dose, he collapsed and required mechanical ventilation (breathing via a machine), artificial feeding and a stay in the ICU for several days. After he woke up, it was discovered that he had suffered significant cognitive deficits and would not be able to work again. The error was acknowledged but the dreams of a stunned family were shattered forever.

The problem: Inadequate review of the records and failure of double-check systems.

Coma

A colleague sent me what he calls a "war story." He was covering a vacationing physician's patients that day. One of the patients on the list was a man who had been unresponsive for several days. As my friend reviewed the records, he discovered that the patient was receiving Percocet, Librium and Elavil for pain, sleep and depression respectively even though he was essentially comatose. All those drugs have sedative properties and should have been withdrawn as soon as feasible. The man, much to his wife's delight, began to wake up as the unnecessary drugs were slowly tapered off.

The problem: Polypharmacy for physician convenience, to avoid numerous nursing calls for agitation, and a lack of effort to understand why the patient was comatose.

Pangs of Conscience

Dr. Van Koinis, a 58-year-old pediatrician and advocate for homeopathic medicine, killed himself in September 2019. His suicide note expressed deep regret over his role in falsifying many documents over a decade so vaccine hesitant parents could "prove" that their children had received the vaccine and attend school. By doing so, he jeopardized the health of others. He did not deny vaccines to families which requested them.[205]

The problem: Succumbing to family pressure to create fraudulent documents and failure to protect children.

Asymmetry

The human body is remarkably symmetrical. New one-sided lumps must be treated with caution. A 49-year-old man was first seen by an APN for a painless lump in his neck and was seen a few days later by a doctor. Both told the patient it was likely a "virus" and not worry because a complete blood count was normal. Several months later, he was seen by a different physician who immediately ordered a biopsy which confirmed cancer. A six-month delay in cancer management can mean the difference between cure and death. Cancer is often painless and blood counts are typically normal in the early stages.

The problem: Anchoring bias about the diagnosis, inadequate reflection about the differential diagnosis.

The operation

A young woman had a colectomy (total removal of the large intestine) for chronic inflammatory bowel disease. The surgeon never referred the patient to a gastroenterology expert to consider medications which are often effective in controlling the disease without surgery. The patient must now live a terrible life with an ileostomy, a procedure where a segment of the small intestine is diverted to the abdominal wall and the contents empty into an external bag. The patient was unaware of the available non-surgical options.

The problem: Lack of knowledge and due diligence in referring to an expert.

Forgiven

The 89-year-old generally healthy man adored the surgeon who intermittently scraped off the patient's small cancerous skin lesions. On one occasion, the surgeon prescribed Bactrim for a skin infection unaware that a much lower dose should be used for the elderly. Several days later, the patient felt tired, confused and was admitted for kidney failure and a dangerously high potassium level caused by high doses of the antibiotic. The surgeon apologized for the error and was forgiven. The patient refused dialysis and died peacefully a few days later.

The problem: Lack of knowledge and failure of a pharmacist to recommend a lower dose.

Drowning the Grandchildren

An elderly woman received an antibiotic called levofloxacin for pneumonia. She became agitated and told me that she had a recurring nightmare that she had methodically drowned all her grandchildren, one at a time, in a bucket of water. A subsequent seizure led to expensive CT scans and an MRI. A brief chart review revealed the diagnosis. Her antibiotic dose was far too high and not adjusted for her age or kidney function. All the symptoms were due to careless dosing. This oversight was costly and caused needless suffering. The patient recovered quickly after the antibiotic was stopped.

The problem: Lack of knowledge and failure of the hospital pharmacy system to prevent this.

Eternal Sleep

An elderly woman developed drowsiness, confusion, tremors, a seizure and an aspiration pneumonia after receiving the antibiotic Cefepime for a urinary infection. Suspecting a stroke, the team ordered a CT scan of the head, but it was obvious to a consultant that she had received excessive doses of Cefepime. Her complications and death were due to an incorrect drug dose. It is a commonly prescribed antibiotic and it is easy to calculate the correct dose. Change occurs at a glacial pace in hospitals but ultimately a system was created which ensured that patients received correct doses in the future. It took five years to change the protocol.

The problem: lack of knowledge and failure of the pharmacy system to prevent this.

Lockjaw

An uninsured farmer came to the hospital for an infected wound on his foot and said he suspected "lockjaw" (tetanus). He received the appropriate injections recommended for this disease. Patients with tetanus die from respiratory failure over days or weeks and must be very carefully monitored, preferably in an intensive care unit. He "looked well" so the team admitted him to a regular hospital bed. Focusing on wound care, the team did not recognize the importance of his new symptoms of difficulty with swallowing food and mild breathing problems which suggested progressive tetanus. Worried about rising bills, he asked to be discharged and died at home a few days from respiratory failure. If he had stayed, he would have incurred unaffordable rising bills which he would need to pay out of pocket. On the other hand, the team failed to recognize the new neurological symptoms and to warn him of the danger.

The problem: lack of knowledge and lapse in clinical judgment-being fooled by a patient "looking well."

A Fatal Omission

Robert Pearl MD, a former CEO of the Permanente part of Kaiser Permanente, one of the largest health care organizations catering to 10 million people, wrote an account of how his father died at a prominent hospital because of a preventable infection after surgery to remove his spleen. It is extremely important and standard practice to give vaccines to patients who are undergoing such surgery because the spleen has a major role in defenses against bacteria. Doctors had forgotten to give his father those vital vaccines before his spleen was surgically removed.²²

The problem: Lack of knowledge or lack of a systemic protocol with a checklist including vaccines

A Nurse charged with reckless homicide

In December 2017, an experienced nurse overrode some safeguards which might have prevented a patient's death at Vanderbilt University Medical Center. Instead of a routine sedative, she gave the patient vecuronium, a paralyzing agent, while the patient was in a body scanning machine for 30 minutes and alone. He became unconscious, suffered a cardiac arrest, had brain damage and died the next day. The event was not reported publicly until Nov 2018 after a CMS inspection uncovered it. The nurse admitted she overrode safeguards (a fairly common problem that accompanies hectic work schedules). Such lapses in safety are mostly related to either poor training or orientation, overwork, distractions, an absence of double-checks within the system and confusion in distinguishing drugs which look alike and sound alike (LASA), are stored close to each other. Why was the patient alone in the MRI suite? Why did the drug error occur? What was the training and enforcement? The leadership accepted no responsibility. Instead, they blamed the nurse for not following procedure and threw her under the bus. She was indicted on a criminal charge of reckless homicide and sentenced to jail. If the patient had done well, no one would have said a word, and the nurse might have continued making the same error. Her punishment was widely condemned by the medical community.[206]

The problem: Inadequate training, overwork, lack of oversight or distraction. One can be sure if this happened once, it had happened before.

Fever

An 84-year-old man was admitted for fevers up to 104 degrees daily for four days. His social history is recorded as "unremarkable" (mostly because no one asked). The medical team wasted thousands of

SICK AND SCARED

dollars in a wild goose chase looking for esoteric causes of fever. When asked, the patient reported that he was an avid outdoorsman who frequently finds ticks on his body. A simple lab test strongly suggested that he had a tick-borne infection called Ehrlichiosis. A better history might have averted this admission. The team's anchoring bias, that an old man would not be active, led to wasted resources and increased cost and delays in care. All he needed was an antibiotic prescription which would cost him $4. His non-physician daughter had suspected a tick-related infection all along!

The problem: Not taking an adequate history and an anchoring bias.

A false note

A family friend read her "intake" note before a procedure was to be performed. The checkmarks indicated that she had a "dependence on illicit drugs." Horrified, the 75-year-old woman demanded that the record be amended immediately. Apparently, a transcribing error occurred when records from another office were incorporated into the hospital chart. This type of misinformation gets "immortalized" in the chart unless corrected quickly.

The problem: Human error in transcribing information.

A Fatal Swap

A 90-year-old woman was brought to the ED for worsening shortness of breath. Pharmacy technicians are trained to prepare a medication list for one patient at a time, print it and then deliver it to the doctors and nurses. A new pharmacy technician prepared and printed medication lists for two patients because she figured she would save time walking to a printer placed in another unit. The two lists were inadvertently swapped, and two patients received wrong medicines. The 90-year-old died four hours later most likely from adverse reactions to the wrong drugs. A quick, unconditional apology was provided to the family acknowledging the institution's mistake. The family would never have known the truth without this disclosure. After initial bewilderment and anger, the family not only forgave the hospital and staff but also made a substantial donation. Workers were retrained to avoid future errors. The printer was brought closer to the workplace.

The problem: Inadequate training, inconvenient location of the printer and lack of double-checks by the nurse and physician.

Polypharmacy

An elderly but alert woman with a doctorate degree was admitted for a urinary tract infection. Within three days, this once vibrant woman became sleepy, incontinent, and unable to get out of bed. She did not recognize family members. The hospitalist, ignoring his professional duty, said he had no time to answer questions from the family because he had "many more patients to see." A family friend, a physician, reviewed the medication list which included a whole slew of unnecessary sedatives and injections for agitation. The family demanded that all medications be stopped except the antibiotic and demanded a discharge before "before they kill her." The patient recovered rapidly at home. Polypharmacy is an American epidemic. Doctors prescribe a pill for every symptom. In this case, if the doctor had taken the time to listen, he might have discovered the reason for the patient's worsening condition.

The problem: Lack of due diligence, courtesy or humility as well as polypharmacy.

Crimes against minorities

When I first arrived in the US in 1971, I heard rumors that black women of childbearing age undergoing any abdominal surgery often had their fallopian tubes tied without consent by white male surgeons "for their own good." That story seemed implausible until I read about the Tuskegee study which was conducted between 1932 and 1972 by the U.S. Public Health Service. Its purpose was to study the natural course of syphilis in untreated black men who were unaware of the diagnosis. None were treated, even after penicillin, an effective treatment, became available in 1945 which resulted in blindness or insanity in some. The research, an eerie reminder of Nazi experiments, was sanctioned by the US government. On May 16, 1997, at 2.26 PM EDT, President Clinton apologized to the eight survivors and the families of all study subjects in The East Room. An excerpt from that speech follows:

"The legacy of the study at Tuskegee has reached far and deep, in ways that hurt our progress and divides our nation. We cannot be one America when a whole segment of our nation has no trust in America. An apology is the first step, and we take it with a commitment to rebuild that broken trust. We can begin by making sure there is never again another episode like this one. We need to do more to ensure that medical research practices are sound and ethical, and that researchers work more closely with communities."

"What was done cannot be undone but we can end the silence. We can stop turning our heads away. We can look at you in the eye, and finally say, on behalf of the American people, what the United States government did was shameful, and I am sorry." The President praised the survivors for their spirit of forgiveness.[207]

The problem: A major systemic defect due to a legalized system of discrimination with little accountability in an era when one human race was considered inferior to another.

2. Harm Due to Lapses in Communication

The Handoff

A doctor admitted a patient for fever on a Friday evening and ordered blood cultures but no antibiotics or fluids. He did not inform the on-call doctor that this patient would need urgent orders and close attention. By the time the nurse called the on-call doctor hours later, it was too late. The patient died from septic shock. The blood cultures revealed a bacterial infection which was essentially untreated at a facility which has all the resources to manage such conditions.

The problem: lack of a handoff, an inefficient and dangerous on-call system with an over-burdened doctor covering 40 patients for six doctors in three hospitals on weekends. The system was designed for physician convenience not for patient safety.

A Missed Dose

A young woman was driving to another state. The abrupt onset of fever, chills, dizziness and a sore throat led to a detour to the nearest ED. The doctor ordered an antibiotic injection before but that did not happen. She was given a prescription, but all pharmacies were closed at that late hour. She was essentially untreated. A few hours later, she returned to the ED in septic shock and died. Tests showed she had a deadly blood stream infection due to "flesh eating bacteria" (group A streptococcus) which should have been treated urgently in the hospital.

The problem: A tragic lapse in communication led to the missed dose which might have saved her life.

A Vacation in New England

A previously healthy woman was admitted with a fever, headaches and confusion. A medical student was the only person who noted "vacation in Maine." Babesia is a parasitic infection transmitted by tick bites and the disease is endemic in Maine. The student's supervisors had not read this note or taken a history themselves. A major teaching opportunity was missed, and the diagnosis was overlooked. A few days later, a very astute laboratory technician found a parasite on a blood smear, which causes a disease known as babesiosis. Inexpensive oral antibiotics cured her, but the entire admission and associated costs could have been averted if there had been a better communication with the patient and within the team.

The problem: Lack of knowledge and missing important epidemiologic information.

SICK AND SCARED

Red-faced

My task was to counsel a new patient whose HIV test was positive. I had done this hundreds of times during my career. I was fully prepared for the wide range of emotions to be expected. I had asked him if he was Mr. X and thought he nodded yes. As I spoke, he started sweating, then hyperventilating and then became hysterical and loud. The charge nurse rushed in and informed me that Mr. X had been moved to a private room. This was Mr. Y. My apology did little to calm him and I felt like an idiot.

The problem: Lack of adherence to established norms for patient identification.

Listen to the Patient

A patient had low-grade fevers for months. His PCP assured him he "looked good" and "not to worry." Several visits and assurances later, the patient sought another opinion. The patient told the consultant that he had a history of a "leaky heart valve" which led to a search for bacteria in the blood and confirmed the diagnosis of endocarditis, a life-threatening infection of a heart valve. He was cured but required antibiotics and heart valve surgery. An earlier diagnosis might have averted surgery.

The problem: Inadequate history and questionable clinical judgment in not investigating further when symptoms continued.

A Cremation

On October 30, 2019, Paul Tyler, a patient in a Pittsburgh nursing home was cremated months before the family knew he had died. The facility did not notify the family and the medical examiner could not find the next of kin. The new facility management refused to answer any further questions.[208]

The problem: Inadequate communication or effort to find the family.

Informed consent

"Informed consent" for surgery is a misnomer. Many patients do not understand the details, potential complications and they do not know which questions to ask. Typically, a surgeon decides that a certain procedure is needed and asks the patient if it is OK to schedule. This is an opportunity to ask questions, to learn more, and to then make a careful, informed decision. These conversations are often perfunctory, and a secretary or nurse asks the patient to sign a document agreeing to a procedure just before surgery. Patients usually sign the papers without any questions based on trust. When things go wrong, the team will use the signed papers to defend themselves.

The problem: doctors often assume that patients understand the nature of the test, procedure and the complications or are too lazy or busy to explain things in plain language. Patients do not want to be "difficult" and keep quiet.

Teeth falling out

Patients sometimes are greatly distressed when they discover that they lost a tooth or two during or after surgery. Tubes and instruments of various types are placed through the mouth for nutrition, ventilation or for diagnostic procedures. These tubes can dislodge already loose teeth, which might get inhaled and lead to aspiration pneumonias. I am aware of several patients who did not know about such complications and were quite annoyed that they were not told about the risk. Thus, physicians doing such procedures should take the time to obtain a proper informed consent.

The problem: Lack of explanation of all the risks especially in people with poor dentition.

The transplant lottery

Two patients in New Jersey, with the same name and similar age, were waiting for a kidney transplant. A mistake resulted in the lower priority patient receiving the kidney first. Luckily, the one who should have received it also received a kidney later.[209]

The problem: Lack of adequate attention to standard identification practices.

A hard pill to swallow

A family friend was discharged after neck surgery. Steroid pills were used to reduce the swelling which occurs after such surgery. He thought the nurse told him to stop the pills after discharge, so he did. A day later, he had trouble swallowing. The family called the surgeon's office and was told by a brusque physician's assistant to "go to the ED if worried." She did not ask any questions to understand what might be happening. We decided to review the written instructions which said to continue the pills. The patient was able to crush a steroid pill and swallow it with great difficulty. He felt well within hours and averted a very costly ED visit.

The problem: Misunderstood discharge instructions or comprehension, busy and brusque PA and patient's delayed review of written discharge instructions.

The scream

A woman was rushed to the OR for an urgent operation. The surgeon made an incision before the anesthesiologist gave his clearance. He had just started anesthetizing the patient and the incision was premature. The patient screamed.

The problem: The surgeon had skipped a vital step in communication and clearance from anesthesia.

The last wish

A chronically ill elderly gentleman signed a consent form for surgery after he fell and broke his femur. Minutes later, he changed his mind and told the Emergency room staff, the hospitalist and nurses that he did not want any surgical intervention. This was not documented in the chart and the surgeon was unaware. The shift changed and the nurse, unaware of the patient's last wishes, sent the patient to the operating room, where he died during unwanted surgery.

The problem: Error in communication and documentation. One team did not communicate with the other.

The DNR order

A terminally ill woman had a living will and a Do Not Resuscitate (DNR) order. A nurse panicked when the patient turned blue and, forgetting that the patient had a DNR order, called a code blue. The code team rushed in, adrenaline flowing, but forgot to ask about the DNR status. Resuscitation efforts failed, as they often do. A shocked family witnessed this war zone with medical paraphernalia strewn across the room as the bruised and battered body was transported to the morgue. Embarrassed team members acknowledged their oversight.

The problem: Ignoring protocol to do a quick check of the chart before proceeding with the CPR.

Dead man talking

One evening I examined a patient who, according to a discharge summary from another hospital, had died three months earlier! The brief discharge note reflected a long and complex hospitalization and stated that "the patient unfortunately succumbed after a stormy hospital course." Here I was, listening to a dead man talking. Perhaps the physician never knew this patient and was dictating on behalf of someone else without checking the chart.

The problem: Doctors often dictate charts in a hurry to satisfy hospital rules and to avoid penalties. Hospitals cannot bill the patient until all chart notes are completed and signed in a timely manner. No one checks the quality and accuracy of discharge notes.

SICK AND SCARED

3. Harm due to Faulty Health Care Systems

The clogged urinary catheter

A patient with a chronic indwelling urinary catheter was admitted to the hospital in shock and died soon after. A nurse at a long-term facility had flushed his clogged catheter using a syringe filled with water. This practice is common and dangerous. If done forcefully, bacteria which are invariably present in such catheters, can migrate up into the kidney and blood stream and result in death from shock. Physicians unaware of this risk may discharge patients with instructions to flush the bladder. A gentle flush is likely not harmful, but it is safer to simply remove and replace a crusted, cracked or clogged catheter.

The problem: A lack of knowledge and failure of systems to abolish such practices.

The dislodged catheter

There is a safety rule that the connections for the catheter used for hemodialysis must always be visible to staff. A drowsy patient, feeling cold, placed a blanket over his arm. The catheter somehow got snagged, fell out and the patient, thought to be sleeping, bled to death. The mattress underneath was soaked with blood. Staff members were rather busy and did not notice the blanket covering the catheter.

The problem: Staff should be vigilant but cannot be expected to keep an eye on each patient constantly. The patient may have been tired, drowsy or unaware that the catheter should be visible. It is unclear how such rare events can be prevented.

The Volunteer

A friend sent me this anecdote. Some years ago, when things were far laxer than they are today, a volunteer, who was not a pharmacist, was helping pharmacy staff fill pill bottles. A cancer patient was prescribed Compazine, which he was to take thrice a day for nausea. His blood tests at the next visit were abnormal suggesting that he might be on a blood thinner. When the physician checked the bottle, it had coumadin, a blood thinner, in it rather than Compazine. Untrained people can be easily fooled because of their unfamiliarity with drug names or because of look-alike and sound-alike drugs. This patient could have bled to death.

The problem: an untrained volunteer could fill bottles without any knowledge of what the dangers might be and unaware of look-alike sound-alike drugs. While done in good faith, it was not good judgment.

Timeliness

Nurse-to-patient ratios determine the timeliness of care. Busy, tired and distracted nurses cannot possibly be perfect. Hospitalized patients rarely receive their medicines, including time sensitive drugs such as insulin, analgesics or antibiotics, at scheduled times. Delays of minutes to hours are common. This hurts patients and makes the hospital look bad.

The problem: if the staffing is inadequate, there is no way for a nurse to do his/her tasks without resorting to short cuts. Many nursing strikes are related to low staffing and salaries.

Bruised babies

A terrible thing happened to Dennis and Kimberly Quaid's twins on November 18, 2007. Writing for the LA times, Charles Orstein wrote: "Before actor Dennis Quaid went to bed Nov. 18, he gave one last call to Cedars-Sinai Medical Center, where his newborn twins were being treated for staph infections.

'Oh, they're fine' Quaid recalled a nurse telling him. 'They're just fine.' They weren't. Earlier that day, nurses had mistakenly given Thomas Boone and Zoe Grace 1,000 times the recommended dose of the blood thinner heparin. About two hours before Quaid's call, nurses had noticed Zoe oozing blood from an intravenous site on her arm and a spot on her heel, state records show. But that night, even as hospital

SICK AND SCARED

staff scrambled to reverse the effects of the heparin, Quaid said, no one notified him or his wife, Kimberly, of the crisis.

The first that Dennis Quaid learned of the medication error was at 6:30 a.m. the next day, he said, when he arrived at the Los Angeles hospital. Treatment decisions had been made without them, he said. "Our kids could have been dying, and we wouldn't have been able to come down to the hospital to say goodbye."

"At the door of the children's hospital room, he said, he was greeted not just by a pediatrician and a nurse but by a representative of the hospital's risk management department." The Quaid family sued the manufacturer for making vials which looked similar, and Cedars Sinai spent millions trying to improve their system.[210]

The problem: Different drugs and vials must not be stored together. Drugs within the same class with different strengths must also be separated and labeled clearly. The labels should be distinctive enough to avoid confusion. There should be double-checks of doses by another individual before the patient receives them.

Food

It is upsetting to see a patient's bed rails up -for safety- and a food tray out of reach or to see the tray contains a huge pile of meat and mush which immediately turns off frail patients with anorexia. Trays often have tasteless or prohibited items. An incredible amount of food is wasted in hospitals. While a hospital does not aspire to have the culinary excellence available on cruise ships, a little more variety to include individual preferences might make the stay happier.

The problem: Hospitals have never aspired to be high-end restaurants. Is that a good strategy for healing or for business?

Instrument count

Instruments, tubes, drains and swabs are sometimes inadvertently left in a body cavity after an operation. There are elaborate systems to prevent this from happening. Yet, at least once or twice a year, most institutions go through the ritual of doing a "root cause analysis" to understand why a sponge, a knife or a drain had been left behind.

The problem: It is almost always due to a failure to follow safety procedures which include checklists and counts before, during and after surgery.

Lack of equipment

A patient had had mild difficulty in swallowing for some years. She was advised to have an endoscopy (inserting a tube with a camera to investigate the esophagus and stomach). While under anesthesia the team realized they needed a pediatric size endoscope, but none was available. The procedure was aborted. She received the full bill anyway (cost of endoscopy, anesthesia, doctor's fee, facility fee, supplies). She then sought a second opinion at another hospital system 50 miles away. After a thorough review, they assured her that a decade old symptom of occasional swallowing difficulty was not a matter for concern. She did not need any further evaluation. She remains well five years later.

The problem: Reflex thinking and scheduling of procedures which might be avoided with a good history as well a systemic issue of not anticipating what tools might be needed.

Burns in the OR

Patients sometimes get deep and painful skin burns because very hot instruments used to stop bleeding from small blood vessels are left on the skin rather than on metal trays. This might indicate a need for better insulated instruments or more vigilance in the operating room.

The problem: Not following established safety protocols.

Dirty Humidifiers

Seven children with cancer have died at the Seattle Children's Hospital since 2001 due to a mold infection. The latest death occurred on Feb 12, 2020. It was mistakenly thought to come from a nitrogen tank. The CDC now believes that the mold had grown in an idle operating room humidifier which had been turned on without cleaning.

SICK AND SCARED

The aerosolized particles containing mold were inhaled by sick children. The hospital was sued and admitted its error in interpreting earlier data. The CEO apologized for the failures and promised to install safer and better systems.[211, 212]

The problem: Erroneous conclusion about the source of infection and inadequate maintenance of machines and pipes on a regular basis.

Contaminated Heater-Cooler Devices

Several patients who received heart surgery developed unusual and often fatal infections involving the blood, the heart valves and other tissues. The worldwide problem was traced to humidifiers manufactured in Germany which were contaminated by the organism, M. Chimera, which grows very slowly and may show up months or years later. Current treatment is not highly effective, and the fatality rates are very high. Numerous patients remain on the at-risk list because they have had such surgery during the period when such machines were used.[213]

The problem: This was an inadvertent contamination by unusual pathogens at a manufacturing facility. It is unclear why this happened, but possibly there was a lapse in the established processes.

The Waiting Room

An elderly man signed into a busy ED saying simply that he felt unwell. The triage nurse took vital signs which were reassuring and directed him to the waiting area. He found a chair behind a vending machine and dozed off. The video cameras do not reach this corner of the ED. He was forgotten in the hustle and bustle and found dead the next morning, in a sitting position with his winter coat and hat still on. Staff members were devastated. How does one prevent such events unless staff members make frequent "rounds" of large waiting rooms?

The problem: There was no system to make sure all patients were accounted for, and the video camera was not able to capture the "blind spot."

Too many X-rays

According to Elizabeth Rosenthal, Florida physicians order x-rays five times more often than physicians in Ohio for Medicare patients.[50] It is highly unlikely that Medicare patients in Florida are much sicker than those in Ohio or that Ohio physicians are doing too few x-rays. While regional differences in test patterns and costs are well known, they do not make scientific sense.

The problem: Too many x-rays suggest insecurity or defensive medicine because of litigation. It is also possible that there are shady practices of referrals and kickbacks.

Too Many Operations

Knee surgery:

Surgeons often perform procedures with dubious value which bring in a lot of money but do not benefit the patient. Whether this is deliberate or not is difficult to gauge. Earlier, I gave the example of my mother who had an arthroscopic exploration of one knee (without benefit) when she really needed bilateral knee replacements. Moseley and his colleagues performed a study to see if sham operations might be just as effective as "real" surgery. Patients with knee pain were randomized in three groups. Group 1 had an incision with simple irrigation of the knee; Group 2 had an incision with no irrigation and group 3 had the full arthroscopic procedure including the incision and scraping of tissue. All patients fared the same.[214] There has been speculation that sham surgery's benefit is a placebo effect. Arthroscopy is clearly useful for traumatic meniscus injuries but not for advanced knee osteoarthritis.

The problem: My reading of this literature suggests that such incremental surgery (arthroscopy followed by knee replacement) simply increases surgical incomes and increases patient risk, harm and cost.

SICK AND SCARED

Spine Surgery:

The rate of spine surgery in the US is five times greater than it is in Canada or Europe, and experts claim that 75% of those are unnecessary. Ask questions. Seek second opinions.50

The problem: Institutions need to develop specific protocols for stepwise interventions for back pain before any spine surgery is done unless it is an emergency. If the decision is left to surgeons, they might lean towards surgery.

Prostate cancer surgery:

To operate or watch: Many men, as they get older, have cancer in the prostate gland. The incidence increases by almost 10% for each decade of life beyond 50. The consensus of experts is that most patients die with the disease and not from it and that many men can be observed without surgery or radiation which can have debilitating side effects such as incontinence and impotence. European surgeons generally offer active surveillance (AS) and avoid surgery. Various criteria are used to determine who can be watched and who must receive immediate treatment. Much angst and cost might be reduced with AS. The US is beginning to tilt in that direction, but there are still far too many surgical excisions.

The Problem: This topic remains controversial. We need better tools to determine who needs surgery and who can be observed. This consensus is developing and will likely lower the cost and harm from such surgery over time.

Caesarian Sections:

I was posted to a remote hospital in Kenya in 1968 and performed scores of C-sections because the local Kikuyu women have a higher rate of pelvic disproportion making vaginal delivery dangerous. These C-sections saved lives. The rate of delivery by C-section in most countries is 10-15% of all deliveries but it is 30% in the US. Possible reasons are that patients want to time their delivery or that obstetricians -who are not in house at night when deliveries commonly occur- perform more C-sections for their own convenience. Hospitals are employing in-house obstetrics hospitalists to lower C –section rates.

The problem: C-sections are convenient for the patient and the surgeon but many of them are unnecessary. Again, protocols must be developed to determine who must undergo a C-section immediately and who should not. Is it appropriate or safe to offer C-sections to women who do not wish to go through labor or want an earlier delivery when there is no increased danger from a vaginal delivery?

4. Other causes of Harm

Reading shadows

I felt an excruciating chest discomfort after I fell and hit the edge of the dresser some years ago. The x-ray was read as normal. I asked for a review and they saw one broken rib. Pressed further, they agreed there were three rib fractures! I also thought there was blood in the chest. The radiologist had misread the x-rays three times.

The problem: Boredom, laziness, exhaustion, distraction or the monotony of work could all explain why a simple chest x-ray would be misread.

Two for One

A patient required urgent gall bladder surgery. The experienced surgeon found matted infected tissues stuck to each other during the operation. The procedure seemed to have gone well until the pathologist reported that the tissue contained the diseased perforated gall bladder stuck to a healthy right kidney.

The problem: People wondered if the surgeon was overworked and exhausted rather than careless.

Cancer chemotherapy

Cancer chemotherapy is complex, dangerous, and it requires meticulous attention to detail. Doses of highly toxic drugs must be calculated carefully and double-checked. The patient must be weighed because doses depend on the actual weight. Is the weight reported in kg or lbs.? Kidney function must be checked regularly otherwise toxic levels may accumulate and damage other organs. These prescriptions are typically scrutinized by highly skilled pharmacists, but if the work volume is high and staffing is inadequate, errors reach the patient with disastrous consequences. I am aware of several events where chemotherapy hurt patients because safeguards, already in place, were not implemented.

The problem: understaffing of pharmacists and their inability to cope with the volume of orders written is a real problem. These pharmacists are an important counter check to doctor's orders which might be inaccurate and dangerous.

Wrong side surgery

I remember well the horror we felt in 1967 when one of our urology professors in medical school removed a healthy kidney instead of the diseased one. He was bright, famous and well liked. Nobody in health care used what is called the universal protocol in those days. The checklist, which is a major component of the protocol, requires that several things be checked off before surgery begins.

Reliance on memory alone is a common cause for mix-ups in surgery, radiological reports and chart notes. When wrong side surgery occurs, it is called a "never or sentinel event" but hospitals do not always report such mistakes. Checklists, time-outs and "universal protocols" should be used to confirm the exact side and site for the surgery. The site should be marked clearly.

The problem: The inadvertent removal of healthy organs, surgery at wrong sites and injections of anesthetic at the wrong site are manifestations of shortcuts, such as not using a checklist or the lack of teamwork. Nurses are often afraid to challenge the surgeon. Each team member must feel empowered to stop the surgery if the wrong side has been selected.

Not asking for Expert Help

Primary care doctors sometimes are too proud to seek help ("I can handle it"), but certain conditions must be managed by experts. The mortality and rate of complications from blood stream infections with "staph" (Staphylococcus aureus) and Candida (a fungus) can be reduced substantially when an expert weighs in. While the desire to cut down on unnecessary consultations is laudable, it is foolish to deny patients the best care possible.

The problem: Arrogance and ignorance are dangerous and equally difficult to manage.

Curbside consults

There are situations where a physician would like to tap the expert's knowledge without creating the formality of the specialist seeing the patient and writing a report. These have become known as "curbside consults." It can be a dangerous practice. Doctors should share their knowledge with colleagues but avoid giving opinions about illnesses without a direct interview and examination of the patient. The information shared is often insufficient, inaccurate or misleading. The consultant may even be quoted in the chart as having recommended a specific treatment, setting up the potential for a malpractice scenario. The ideal response should be "this sounds complicated. It would be better if I could examine the patient and review all records." It is much safer for the patient.

The problem: Lack of awareness of the unintended consequences of curbside consults. It is an unsafe practice and dangerous for the doctor who seeks a curbside consultation, to the one who agrees to offer curbside advice consult and to the patient.

White coat hypertension

Patients in the hospital are anxious, and their blood pressure (BP) may fluctuate greatly. When a nurse calls a doctor because a patient's blood pressure is too high, the typical response is to prescribe a BP medicine or add medicine to what is already being given. This is a bad practice and potentially harmful. A better plan is to ask if the pressure was measured correctly with the right-sized cuff. The smart physician would ask that the BP be checked again when the patient is calm and relaxed.[215]

SICK AND SCARED

The problem: it is easier to prescribe something immediately rather than ask the nurse to check the BP again and call back. More often it is out of concern for the high BP and possible harm to the patient. Data suggests it is safe to take the watch and wait approach.

The Annual Physical

The honest PCP will not recommend preventive services like "executive physicals" offered by the nation's top hospitals, for profit and prestige. The affluent and worried-well pay thousands of dollars, out of pocket, for tests which no one thinks are necessary or appropriate. These annual tests set a bad precedent and are wasteful.[216]

The US Preventive Services Task Force (USPSTF) issues guidelines and ranks a variety of tests from A-I based on evidence. These differ a bit from European or Canadian guidelines, but most agree on what is unnecessary. A recent study reported that the nation's top 50 hospitals routinely offered tests which were rated D (not recommended) or I (insufficient evidence). Only 2 of 16 tests had a strong A recommendation, 2 had B or moderate and 2 had C (selective) ratings.[217]

The problem: Simply stated, it is institutional, or physician greed which preys on the gullible and wealthy. This is dishonest, even if the "customer" is paying out of pocket. This is not health care. It is a transfer of wealth.

Sins of Medicine

Another problem in the era of specialization is that physicians seem to order a test for every symptom rather than take the time to figure out how all the symptoms might be interconnected and caused by one disease. Brendan Reilly writes about a man with benign paroxysmal positional vertigo (BPPV) who got a hurried history followed by numerous tests/ imaging from many specialists. This was followed by a bill for $74,542. If the first MD had "googled" the symptoms, BPPV would have shown up as the most likely diagnosis, requiring no further diagnostics. The patient's 30-year-old niece, a physician, suspected the diagnosis as soon as he told her the symptoms. BPPV, a condition where patients fall after assuming certain positions, requires no further testing or treatment.[218]

This type of evaluation and referral pattern is common. It is thoughtless, automatic and robotic. Clinical stupidity (the opposite of commonsense) and "sloth" (laziness) were two of the seven sins of medicine described by the physician Richard Asher in a lecture delivered in London, UK in 1949.[219]

The problem: A good primary care physician with enough time –and commonsense- would be able to consider all possibilities without so much waste and worry.

Bill Collection

A hospital in Carlsbad, New Mexico not only overcharged patients but also was ruthless in asking collection agencies to file lawsuits to collect the debts. Judges- some of whom had been sued as well- had no choice but to garnish the wages of people who could ill afford a pay cut. Families were ruined. The same services in nearby Roswell Hospital cost far less.[13]

The problem: Different pricing in nearby hospitals for the same services, heartless collection policies and a legal system which allows the wages of the poor to be garnished.

A woman in Alabama dropped her insurance because her business was struggling, but she subsequently had to undergo an emergency appendectomy in May 2016. The bill was $ 52,000. The Flowers Hospital in Alabama gave her a "discount" and reduced the bill to $31,000 (Medicare allows $5,800.00 for this procedure). She paid $25 each month for three years. About this time, the hospital sued her for $37,000- the full amount plus interest. She told her husband "I wish you'd have let me die" so "you would not be going through this."[220]

The problem: Simply said, this is a cruel system where an uninsured person is asked to pay far more than an insured person would.

SICK AND SCARED

The Lexington Medical Center in West Columbia, SC is being sued for allegedly seizing tax refunds of people to cover overdue bills after they had filed for bankruptcy, a practice forbidden by federal law. The medical center collected $15.6 million in 2015 and $19.2 million in 2017 using such tactics.[221]

The problem: skirting federal law.

The HIV Story

Our government did little to help people with HIV disease because of overt and occult bias against gay men who were most affected. It was called the "gay disease" which some felt was "divine retribution" for a sinful life. That launched an activist movement which led to some progress, but effective drugs remained extremely expensive and unaffordable until later. There is never any justification ever to punish people who are already suffering from a life-threatening illness.

The frustration, anger and the emotional harm caused were described by the late Randy Shilts in his book *"And the Band Played On."*[222] It was not just lack of government support but also a resistance within the medical community of surgeons who would not operate on these people, and physicians who did not want gays and drug users scaring away mainstream patients from their waiting rooms.

The pre-1990 days of AIDS were a long way from medicine's finest hour. The affected people also included drug users who had little public sympathy. That changed when hemophiliacs such as Ryan White and people just going to the dentist, such as Kimberly Bergailis, got infected and died. The empathy for the two (labeled "innocent victims") was in stark contrast to the others who were being punished for their lifestyle choices.

The problem: this is a question for society to answer. Are we our brother's keepers?

Patent Violations

In an era when HIV treatment costs exceeded $20,000 annually, and the US government dragged its feet, CIPLA, an Indian company stepped up to manufacture generic versions of US drugs and sold them for an annual price of $160 still making huge profits. CIPLA claimed it had not violated any patent because it "tweaked" the manufacturing process." Countless lives were saved in resource-poor nations. American pharmaceutical companies, which had developed these very profitable drugs at great cost, understandably cried foul. Society must answer two questions. Is it morally justifiable to withhold life saving drugs for profit? Is it unethical to steal formulae to save lives? What would you do?

The problem: Could US companies have partnered with government and other companies to find an affordable treatment while still making a lot of money? The answer is clearly yes.

Vaccine Hesitancy

Dr. Andrew Wakefield, a British doctor and his colleagues, published a fraudulent paper in 1998 alleging a link between childhood vaccines and autism in a study of 12 children.[223] Several of the original authors expressed regret about the fabricated data and asked to withdraw their names from the citation. Wakefield had received payments from lawyers for families which were suing vaccine makers. Subsequent large studies could not confirm Wakefield's findings and the paper was retracted by Lancet in 2010. But the harm had already been done. Vaccine hesitancy led to outbreaks of measles, a lethal disease which killed 140,000 children last year.

The vaccination rate for influenza, a disease which kills thousands, is just around 50% in the US. The Wakefield paper was a huge setback to vaccination, and it caused great harm to science, resulting in hundreds of thousands of patients acquiring infections that could have been avoided.[224]

SICK AND SCARED

Anti-vaccination groups have threatened to kill doctors who criticize them. MedPage Today reported the online bullying of a physician who posted a TikTok song "Cupid Shuffle" about the benefits of vaccination and how it does not cause autism. The doctor, a pediatrician in Cincinnati, was surprised by 50,000 views and its being shared it on Twitter. Members of anti-vaccination groups then mounted a coordinated assault on her online reputation. One threatening message stated, "Dead Doctors Don't Lie."[225] A famous proponent of vaccines, who gave a talk at my hospital, asked us to arrange security for him.

People often invoke religious beliefs to reject a vaccine. But religions came much before vaccines were discovered. No religion forbids protecting the young and vulnerable. An employee at the Philadelphia Children's Hospital was fired for refusing to take a flu shot after doing so for many years. She sued alleging that it violated her "African Holistic healthy Lifestyle." A US court ruled her lifestyle belief was not a religion or religious mandate and dismissed the case.[226]

The problem: Fear of vaccines must be overcome with information and education. Each health care worker can become an advocate by setting an example.

Herbal Medicines

Just because it is labeled herbal, "natural" and is widely advertised, does not make it safe. The FDA has little oversight over such drugs and the ingredients are often unknown. There are reports of poisoning from toxic ingredients contained within, including lead. Some unregulated manufacturers incorporate valium, steroids or pain killers within the capsule. No wonder patients feel better! Mega vitamin claims are unsupported by evidence. And some are dangerous.

The problem: this is an unregulated industry. Oversight of a multi-billion-dollar business is going to be difficult. People afraid of modern medicine will always look for something "natural" even if it is contaminated and dangerous.

Going Generic

Generics, said to have similar bio-potency to brand names, are less expensive. Pharmacies charge much more if you ask for a brand name. Recently there have been many recalls due to traces of carcinogens in some generics including blood pressure pills. There is also concern about the potency, quality control and hygiene at overseas manufacturing plants which rarely get spot inspections. Most of these drugs are manufactured in India and China with inadequate oversight. When inspections do occur, the plants get advance notice and have time to "clean up their act." The FDA, which does have jurisdiction over drugs which are imported to the US, does not conduct surprise inspections overseas. Katherine Eban, in her provocative new book, calls generics *Lies in a Bottle*.[227]

Rosemary Gibson and Janardan Prasad Singh, in their book *China Rx: Exposing the Risks of America's Dependence on China for Medicine* write that the US is now so dependent on China for the ingredients used in generic drugs that it is a national security risk. Additionally, they state that the FDA does not have either the will or capacity or both to inspect Chinese plants.[228]

The problem: We are stuck with generic drugs. Most are likely safe and effective. The exceptions are cautionary tales, but I am uncertain what the options are.

Over-the-Counter Drugs

A young professor took an over-the-counter drug called ibuprofen in increasing doses for severe back pain. When it did not help, he went to an urgent care center where he was told to take ibuprofen in higher doses. A few days later, still suffering significant back pain, he went to the local ED. There, he was told that he may have passed a kidney stone and that his blood test showed a "slight kidney problem." He was asked to follow up with his private doctor in 2-5 days. Being new to the area, he had not had the time to find one. Multiple practices were "closed" to new patients. Finally, he got an appointment with a hospital clinic through my intervention. Meanwhile, he kept taking ibuprofen for the lingering back pain. By the time he got to the clinic, he had full blown kidney failure and was admitted.

The kidney failure was due to the over-the-counter ibuprofen. Fortunately, he improved without the need for dialysis. Drugs in this category, the so called nonsteroidal anti-inflammatory drugs (NSAIDs) include Motrin, Aleve, naproxen and ibuprofen, frequently cause of kidney failure and life-threatening bleeding from the stomach, especially in the elderly.

The problem: Commercials glorify these drugs without warning of the major dangers from OTC drugs. We see the complications regularly in hospitals all over the country.

Fairs for the faithful

Places of worship often serve their communities by bringing in nurses and doctors to screen patients for diseases like hypertension, diabetes, high cholesterol, breast cancer, and to counsel about nutrition and lifestyle changes.

But some health fairs have become recruiting grounds for vascular specialists (cardiologists, surgeons and interventional radiologists) who con people into unnecessary operations to open "leg blockages" using catheters. Representatives for sleazy practices do "screening tests" at no cost, and then entice patients to undergo further tests and/or surgery. Patients with claudication, a painful cramp in the thigh or calf on exertion, are a legitimate reason for such operations. So, they ask patients if they ever get leg pain. Since every human being on this planet has occasional leg pain, this is listed as "claudication." The victims are often poor minorities on Medicaid. Church pastors, unaware of the deception, think they have done a great public service for their constituents. The vascular specialists are laughing all the way to the bank.[13]

The problem: Physicians taking advantage of trusting uninformed patients for personal gain. Such practices are unethical. The only way to stop the scam is to bring it to public attention, get state boards involved and find a way to standardize care protocols based on sound science.

Cardiology scams

I am aware of patients who receive annual or biannual echocardiograms and stress tests (costing thousands) because they had a stent placed in their coronary arteries many years ago. These tests are unnecessary if patients have no new symptoms. It is a money-making scheme for the doctors.

The problem: Colleagues are reluctant to identify these bad practices whether done out of ignorance or greed.

***

How do we tackle these issues? I review some strategies to prevent or reduce harm in Part 8.

PART 8

THE JOURNEY TO ZERO HARM

It is clearly unreasonable to expect that doctors will never make a mistake. Overworked, tired and sleep deprived individuals will make even more mistakes. The hospital's culture determines how errors are managed. If leaders are shortsighted and choose to punish people for mistakes, the workers will quickly learn that it is unsafe to report their errors.

When a patient is harmed, great institutions try to understand what happened, why it happened and what can be done to prevent such mistakes in the future. Their workers feel confident that their reports are being reviewed and will contribute to future efforts to improve safety. Such institutions can coach people out of bad habits and behaviors. Reckless behavior from health care workers is rare and requires prompt punishment.

Millions of people get safe and excellent care everyday even though the overall health system is fragmented and disjointed. However, even a low rate of errors harms or kills thousands of patients. It is only when one reviews aggregate data for large populations that the full picture becomes clear. I have been surprised at the number of physicians, nurses and physician assistants who seem to be unaware of extent of health care related harm. Even seasoned physicians have raised an eyebrow when provided with the data.

The concept of zero hospital-acquired harm, when first introduced, was labeled a crazy, unrealistic and foolish dream of idealists living in a medical Utopia. The skeptics said some harm is inevitable when we do invasive procedures or use drugs with known adverse effects. And they are right. There is inherent risk in every treatment and procedure. Chemotherapy to destroy cancerous cells inevitably damages healthy ones too. Killing harmful bacteria with antibiotics invariably results in collateral damage to "good bacteria" which help to protect us. All surgical procedures carry some risk of bleeding or infection. Catheters placed in a large vein are life savers for critically ill patients, but even with proper technique, the surgeon may hit the lung while trying to insert a central catheter. Air may leak out into the space outside the lung and cause a dangerous situation.

But the skeptics missed the point. The real aim of Zero Harm was to try to control *preventable harm;* to embark on a journey to learn what was possible. Given the high stakes, was it not worth trying?

Hospitals in the past had a lukewarm commitment to safety. There were very few systematic interventions targeted towards the reduction of harm. Infection control programs and other safety programs were underfunded and understaffed even though the cost of hospital-acquired infections and harm is extremely high. Those administrative decisions were short sighted and hurt patients.

The publication of the Institute of Medicine (IOM) report suggested that the risk of harm and death in the hospital had been vastly underestimated.[76] The sensational monograph was a wake up call. A greater effort was then made to reduce errors. Specialists and administrators were hired in large numbers. Yet, twenty years after the IOM report, it appears patients face higher risks of death and permanent injury safety today.

Change comes at a glacial pace in hospitals. The malaise seems built into the DNA of institutions. Too often there is a lot of talk but little action. Red tape and "Town and gown" issues impede progress. I recall working on a safety policy for one year with dozens of reform minded leaders but our recommendation was shot down by the decision making body in 5 minutes with little discussion. They felt the harm was rare and did not need another policy. In my mind, even one preventable death is one too many. Indeed, most of the people who voted "nay" were following the "leader" like sheep and had not even read the policy!

Reform measures gather speed when there is bad publicity, financial loss, threat of lawsuits or when an external agency threatens penalties. In this section I wish to describe how and why hospitals are finally moving in the right direction. The reasons for that change are:

- The creation of infection control "bundles" by the Centers for Disease Control (CDC).
- Wider use of checklists.
- The quest for recognition as top hospitals in a highly competitive health care market.
- Requirement by the CMS for public reporting of harm on the website Hospital Compare.
- Financial penalties and incentives imposed by the CMS for harm rates worse or better than national averages.*

*Note: Dissenters might quote the paper by Hsu et al. that reported[229] that the penalties had little effect on hospital acquired infection rates and the gap between safety-net hospitals and non-safety-net hospitals remained wide. The authors concluded that such penalties punish safety-net hospitals financially since their patients are usually uninsured, are on Medicaid and are sicker than wealthier insured patients. These results could have been affected by the way the authors measured the differences. For example, they used infection rates from the National Hospital Safety Network (NHSN) rather than the standardized infection risk adjusted ratios reported by the CMS, and there were also definition changes for the infections and other potential confounding factors during the study period).

Regardless, I know that hospitals fear penalties and the loss of reputation and work hard to avoid them. I am convinced that the carrot (save money by reducing harm and avoiding penalties) and stick (lose money and be embarrassed) approach made a difference in at least some hospitals. I doubt that a purely volunteer effort without oversight from the CMS or the Joint Commission would have succeeded.

I will describe how we can prevent harm from infections and other system issues next.

Prevention of Infections

Vaccines

In the late eighteenth century, Edward Jenner observed that milkmaids did not get smallpox, a disease that killed so many. He suspected that they were immune because of previous exposures to infected cows. In 1796, he took material from a cowpox pustule and injected James Phipps and other children to see if he could protect them. Critics, especially the clergy, claimed it was "repulsive and ungodly" to inoculate someone with material from a diseased animal. A cartoon showed people who had been vaccinated sprouting cow's heads.[230] Jenner's experiments led to the concept of vaccination; a word derived from the Latin *vacca* (cow). In 1977, the WHO announced that smallpox had been eradicated worldwide thanks to the work of the late Dr. Donald Henderson whom I had the privilege to meet twice. Countless lives were saved.

Hemophilus influenza (H. flu) meningitis, a bacterial infection, used to kill 12,000 American children annually and maim many more but is now so rare that most medical students have not seen a case.

Except for a few cases in Pakistan, Afghanistan and Nigeria, polio has been eradicated from the world, saving thousands from the "iron lung" and crippled limbs. (There have been a few cases related to the "live" vaccine elsewhere which resulted in recommendations to use a "killed" vaccine in the US).

The influenza virus vaccine is not perfect but multiple calculations suggest that even a low efficacy vaccine saves thousands of lives due to "herd immunity." Many more would be saved if our vaccination rates improved. Only 37% of adults and 59% of children in the US received

SICK AND SCARED

the flu shot during the 2018-2019 season. Those who reject the vaccine imperil the lives of others. Hospitals are making vaccination mandatory so that sick unvaccinated employees do not transmit the disease to patients and to each other.

The Ebola virus epidemic, first identified in 1976 in Congo, ravaged West African nations including Sierra Leone in 2014-5 and other countries in the region. My friend, the late Dr. William Close, published a personal account of the epidemic when he was in Belgian Congo, now called the Democratic Republic of Congo.[231] Ebola returned with a vengeance recently. Dozens of physicians and many nurses became ill or died caring for patients. But this time, scientists were able to develop and distribute a highly effective vaccine and treatment within a short time despite the challenging and sometimes hostile geopolitical realities of that volatile region.

Vaccine hesitancy has led to recent outbreaks of measles in the US. Why does the richest nation on the planet have so many cases of a preventable disease? Measles killed 140,000 patients worldwide last year. Pneumonia, encephalitis and death are particularly common in malnourished children with measles. Who will protect little children if their parents and our health system do not do so?

As I write this, the world is experiencing turmoil due to a novel coronavirus, the cause of COVID-19 disease, which has infected millions across the globe and killed hundreds of thousands. Economies are devastated. Commerce is halted. Nations are at a standstill. Borders are closed. Planes are parked on runways. Rising shortages, high prices and record unemployment have ruined families. Millions of Americans lost their health insurance because they were laid off. How can this be in a nation as rich as ours?

What is obvious is that we were far too late in addressing the emergency. The nation failed to unite and enforce simple measures such as wearing masks consistently, cleaning hands frequently and keeping a social distance from others. The only reason for the disarray was that some politicians interfered with the work of scientists and epidemiologists and set a bad example for our citizens.

Once again, science will come to the rescue. Scientists have already identified the new virus, sequenced its genome and have potential treatments in the pipeline. The race to produce an effective vaccine has become an international priority, and we are getting closer with several candidate vaccines. I fear another campaign by anti-vaccination groups could derail the progress. Additionally, the contradictory messages from politicians and scientists may create doubt whether the speedy development of a vaccine is driven by a political agenda or with scientific rigor.

Streptococcus pneumonia vaccines are highly effective in preventing lethal lung infections in those at high risk. The vaccine is recommended for children under 2, adults over 65 and some special groups in between. The vaccination rate for adults older than 65 is under 70%.

We know that sexual activity is common in adolescents. The human papilloma virus (HPV) can cause oral, anal and genital cancer in men and women. Seventy-nine million people are already infected in the US, and 14 million acquire a new infection annually. We have three highly effective vaccines, so it is shocking that only 50% of young people at risk are vaccinated.

One third of all elderly patients will suffer from a bout of herpes zoster (shingles). It is an extremely painful, pustular rash usually on the chest wall but may also affect the forehead and the eyes as well. It is usually unilateral but may be disseminated. A terrible sequel to this rash may be a lifelong pain along the nerve roots where the virus causes havoc. It makes adults cry. We now have a two-dose vaccine called *Shingrix* which is 90% effective in preventing shingles and its cost is covered by Medicare. All people over the age of 50 should take it.

Vaccines have saved millions of lives. How do we convince vaccine deniers that vaccines are generally safe? We must also provide easier access to vaccines during primary care visits, at Farmers Markets, at grocery stores and in places of worship. Vaccine manufacturers should be immune from lawsuits if they launched their product in good faith and with scientific backup. They provide an overwhelming public service. And all vaccines should be free for everyone. Once the benefits of a vaccine on public health are established, the insurers who pay for its availability and administration invariably include these, not only as insurance benefit, but encouragement for their beneficiaries to get vaccinated.

The overall adherence to guidelines established by The Advisory Committee on Immunization Practices (ACIP) is just around 58% for the age group 19-35 months.[232] We can do better.

Hand Hygiene (HH)

This is an excerpt from an essay I wrote for FOCUS, a magazine of Christiana Care, Delaware in February 2014.

"In 1847, when the germ theory was still unknown, Ignaz Semmelweis demonstrated that cleaning hands before delivering babies dramatically reduced the number of maternal deaths due to infections. Almost 170 years later, most American hospitals have hand hygiene rates lower than 50%. Why should that be so? We have the most expensive health care in the world and certainly no shortage of soap, running water or alcohol gel. But the message that 'dirty hands kill' seems to have fallen on deaf ears."

Midwives who used a caustic solution to clean their hands had far fewer infections than medical students who delivered babies after doing autopsies but without cleaning their hands. Semmelweis surmised that something from those bodies was causing the deaths. He was shunned, ridiculed, denied promotions, developed dementia and ultimately died in an asylum where he was beaten to death.

Observations show hand hygiene (HH) rates between 20-60% despite great efforts to change the behavior. Most experienced infectious disease experts are baffled by these dismally low rates and are skeptical about claims of great success with intermittent education, signs and slogans. Robert Weinstein MD from Chicago, a friend and pioneer in the field of infection prevention, colorfully suggests that the hands of health care workers are covered by a "fecal patina." Would you eat a slice of pizza if your hands were covered with feces?

HH is cheap, easy and highly effective. Infection prevention manuals emphasize its importance, but hospitals rarely coach those who forget to wash their hands or enforce the behavior. Our behavior might change If patients were to drop dead immediately after a "dirty" touch. Since the infections occur days or weeks later, there is little to connect a specific health care worker to that event. Thus, there is no sense of personal guilt or accountability.

When employees are asked if they routinely wash hands, they say it is "most of the time." But those self-perceptions are very inaccurate. When asked why they do not or did not wash hands, they give multiple answers: "I forgot; the sinks are too far away; the alcohol gel dispensers are not placed conveniently; the soap or gel is rough on my skin; I was in a hurry; I was not planning to touch anything or anyone; it was an emergency; they could not see me washing hands inside the room" etc. There is some validity to the argument that there is not enough time to perform HH, especially for nurses who may enter patient rooms very frequently.

Reliance on posters, signs and clever inspirational messages is ineffective. In a series of experiments in the 1920s at the Western Electric Hawthorne Factory in Illinois, it was discovered that work output at an industrial plant improved when workers knew they were being observed. Many believe that this "Hawthorne Effect" was due to the fear of supervisors but that was just part of it. The increase in productivity was driven also by the interest the supervisors took in the workers. Infection prevention departments must deploy more people where the patients are instead of being cooped up behind computer screens gathering more data about missed opportunities.

Numerous electronic monitoring devices (flashing lights, badges which register data, videos, gadgets which are "awakened" when the faucet is turned on) have been used. These devices generate much data. But few systems use the data to identify and coach frequent offenders. I believe coaching can be an effective way to change behavior. Another possibility is that patients can become more assertive and demand hand hygiene before and after every encounter with health care workers.

SICK AND SCARED

Some hospitals have a sign in patient rooms saying something to the effect that if you didn't see people clean their hands, don't let them touch you.

HH rates are typically monitored and reported internally by hospitals. The reports greatly exaggerate the true HH rates. The false rates lead to a sense of security and nothing gets changed. I believe that regulatory bodies need to do a lot more surprise spot inspections to learn the truth. We delude ourselves into believing things which we know are not true. And they hurt patients.

Central Line Infections

Central catheters (tubes placed in the neck, chest or groin to deliver intravenous medications and or fluids to hospitalized patients) save many lives. But bacteria, which are always present on the skin, can enter the puncture site and cause disastrous infections of the blood stream. For years, everyone accepted the terrible harm as inevitable. Dr. Peter Pronovost, an intensivist and anesthesiologist, had embarked on the safety journey after a disastrous outcome for a child he had cared for at Johns Hopkins. Indeed, some of the greatest crusaders in the safety movement have been either physicians who inadvertently hurt their patients, or family members whose relatives suffered grievous harm in a hospital. He was involved in the Keystone project in Michigan to reduce central line infections. It was an important step forward. Investigators in 108 ICUs were able to reduce central line infection rates by 66% during the 18-month study.[233]

They followed the "bundle," a set of guidelines created by the Centers for Disease Control (CDC) which consists of asking questions about the following: the need for a central catheter versus the employment of a peripheral line; the preference of a safer site (the neck or chest) as a preferred location rather than the microbiologically dirtier groin; the insistence upon hands being washed; the employment of barrier precautions (gloves, gowns, masks, large drapes); and importantly, the assurance that each team member is empowered to halt the procedure for any violations of the protocol.

A decade ago, a newspaper published a very embarrassing and damaging article about the high rate of central line infections at a local hospital. The publicity forced the hospital to follow already established guidelines. Prior to that, it was "business as usual." A major initiative was launched, in collaboration with Dr. Peter Pronovost, to reduce infection rates. The disciplined effort was successful with many units reporting zero infections. That success has been sustained over the years. The skeptics were silenced.

It is possible to get to zero. CMS now reports such data for all hospitals quarterly in the Hospital Compare web site.

Sternal Wound infections

Surgeons cut open the breastbone (sternum) when they perform a coronary artery bypass or when they replace or repair a heart valve. A sternal wound infection causes a collection of pus, a flail chest, great pain and suffering and sometimes death. These infections used to keep infectious disease doctors very busy and brought in revenue. It was a tragic way to earn a living.

At one hospital, the rates began to plummet after the arrival of a new surgeon. When asked about it, he modestly said it was a "bunch of things." What he had done was to introduce and enforce best practices. There were strict rules for antisepsis, timely prophylactic antibiotics, shorter operating room time and reduced blood transfusions. Infection rates for sternal would infections at that hospital have hovered around zero for several years now. Soon after, CMS introduced financial penalties and requirements for public reporting.

Urinary Catheters

Urinary catheters allow external bacteria to enter the bladder. It is inevitable. Some patients are simply colonized without any symptoms. Other get mild catheter-associated urinary tract infections (CAUTI) involving the bladder or they are afflicted with severe kidney or blood stream infections. Some will die. Patients with neurologic conditions such as spinal injury and paralysis unfortunately may need long term catheters if techniques such as intermittent catheterization cannot be used.

There are steps one can take to reduce the infection rates. Obviously, the best strategy would be to avoid unnecessary insertions. When the catheter must remain for a long period, it is standard practice to use a "closed drainage" system and ensure the free and unobstructed flow of urine. Some are using expensive catheters coated with silver or antibiotics (doxycycline and rifampin) which can delay infections.

In 1990, years before it was mandated, the infection control team at a 300 bed VA hospital created a list of appropriate indications for catheter use based upon the available literature. All staff members agreed to abide by the guideline. The infection control nurse made daily rounds on each unit to ask how many patients had indwelling catheters and why they had been inserted. The nurse or I would then urge the doctor to remove catheters which did not fall within the guidelines. For the most part, they agreed to do so. This simple method took just a few minutes each day and quite possibly prevented many infections and saved some lives.

Twenty-five years later in 2015, the CMS required all hospitals to follow urinary tract infection prevention guidelines and assessed penalties for outliers. The guidelines were almost identical to what we used in the VA in 1990. CAUTI also became a publicly reportable infection. Prior to the CMS rules, many private hospitals had little data or oversight over CAUTI. Often, they did not even know how many patients had catheters and how many were unnecessary. Rates at many institutions for CAUTI are close to zero now.

Surgical Wound Infections

A few patients will develop post-operative infections regardless of the efforts made to prevent them. The rates vary based upon the type of surgery and the patient's body habitus. A disciplined approach with teamwork can keep infections within or lower than nationally accepted numbers. This data is reported at the CMS website Hospital Compare as well as certain surgical registries. I have seen surgeons and infection prevention staff get together to brainstorm how to reduce rates especially when they exceed certain thresholds. This type of collaboration was unusual in the past.

Patients may be asked to clean themselves with a cloth containing antiseptic solutions like chlorhexidine before surgery. They will be asked to use depilatory creams or clippers rather than shave the surgical site because the razor can cause little nicks and cuts allowing bacteria to enter. The team must ensure that a single dose of a prophylactic antibiotic is administered in a timely manner before surgery. And if surgery is prolonged, a second dose of the same antibiotic is given. With the CMS reporting requirements, it becomes obvious what type of operation is causing more infections than average, allowing the hospital to take remedial measures.

Clostridioides Difficile (C diff) Diarrhea

The gastrointestinal tract has billions of "good" bacteria which protect us. Antibiotics given for any reason can kill the good ones and allow "bad" bacteria like C difficile to proliferate. They can live in the gut without causing any harm, but some species produce a toxin which causes severe diarrhea and even death. In 2001, a virulent form of toxin was identified after an outbreak in Quebec. It spread rapidly throughout North America. The death rates approached 17% especially in the elderly and caused recurrent infections in 20-40% of the survivors. The treatment was to use rather expensive antibiotics for prolonged periods. This treatment was often unsuccessful. For those who failed all antibiotics efforts, many institutions, including my own, began a fecal transplant program (with cure rates of 90%). The idea was to replace the bad C diff with good gut bacteria from a healthy stool donor. We also used machines which emit ultraviolet light and kill C diff in rooms used by infected patients.

Our rates are not down to zero yet, but we have made progress. Success will be tied to better hand hygiene and lesser use of antibiotics.

SICK AND SCARED

Our institution produced an educational video in 2013, titled "Seven Flowers," to illustrate the severe harm to patients. It was the brainchild of Timothy Hennessy, an internal medicine physician, who was devastated when one of his patients developed C. diff and died from it. In the video, a calm and forgiving family member stated, "it is sad to think that our mother died simply because someone did not wash their hands." We used the phrase "no exceptions, excuses or exemptions" to promote hand hygiene. The video is available on YouTube.[234]

Spores of C. diff are ubiquitous in hospital environments and tough to kill. The unwashed hands of employees are effective vectors of these spores to susceptible patients. Isolation of patients, terminal cleaning of rooms with disinfectants and ultraviolet lights can help reduce the risk as well as meticulous surface cleaning with approved antiseptic agents. The CMS has the same reporting rules for C diff and penalties for being outliers.

Pneumonia

Patients are at risk for pneumonia in the hospital. Several interventions are effective in preventing such pneumonias. They include (1) raising the head of the bed to 30% or higher to prevent aspiration of stomach contents into the lungs. It is a simple measure which costs nothing (2) avoiding acid-reducing medicines called proton pump inhibitors (like Nexium or Prevacid) which neutralize stomach acid necessary to kill bacteria (3) getting vaccinated against pneumococcal pneumonia and influenza.

Antibiotic Misuse

Foreign countries are severely criticized for allowing people to buy antibiotics over the counter like candy. However, we are not doing much better in the USA. While we cannot buy antibiotics without a prescription in the US, it turns out that almost 50% of our antibiotic use is inappropriate. Cost and side effects aside, we may reach a point when indiscriminate use creates super mutant resistant bacteria which cannot be killed by our current cache of drugs.

Why does this happen? Most American doctors and APNs are inadequately trained in antibiotic use. Yet anyone with a certificate on the wall feels he/she is an expert. We do not let clinicians just out of medical school prescribe cancer drugs because of the potential for severe immediate harm. But any clinician can prescribe antibiotics. Harm occurs when antibiotics kill good bacteria and permit resistant bacteria to flourish. This creates the conditions suitable for C diff. and other resistant pathogens. Infections due to resistant bacteria are tough to treat, and the pipeline for new antibiotics has dried up.

Manufacturers have little interest in producing drugs which are used intermittently for short periods. It is just not as profitable as selling drugs which are needed lifelong (like insulin for diabetes, or medicines for blood pressure and high cholesterol). There is no financial impetus for finding new antibiotics.

The implementation of programs like "Choosing Wisely" has been spotty and halfhearted although there are some bright spots especially among pediatricians. Doctors need to get smarter, know their limitations and control their prescribing habits. Patients and families can help by (1) not demanding antibiotics for indications such as common colds or sinus headaches (2) questioning the pros and cons of each prescription and (3) not writing terrible online reviews when they are denied an antibiotic.

Infections due to the Hospital Environment

Hospitals are inherently dangerous places for those whose immune systems don't work well. The deadliest bacteria known to us are found here. If the environment is not maintained properly, these places of healing can become killing fields. Let us look at a few examples:

SICK AND SCARED

Legionnaire's Disease

The outbreak of Legionnaires Disease in July 1976 at the Bellevue-Stratford Hotel on Broad Street in Philadelphia killed 34 and sickened 200. It was determined to be due to bacteria from a cooling tower nineteen floors above street level. The mist from this system had fallen to the ground and was sucked in the lobby through a vent on the ground floor. Apparently, the same infection had sickened three members of the Independent Order of Odd Fellows who attended a convention in 1974 at the same hotel. The elderly and smokers were particularly vulnerable. The newly identified clusters of unusual pneumonias were newsworthy but in retrospect the offending microbe was already known as the cause of Pontiac fever in Michigan where several patients had developed fever, sore throat and body aches without pneumonia. There have been several outbreaks in or near hospitals as well.

It is known that legionella bacteria are found in many large water systems and in inadequately maintained air-conditioning equipment. Ola Ruark RN, an infection prevention nurse, and I collaborated in a national study with Dr. Victor Yu, one of the world's foremost experts on legionella, (then at the Pittsburgh VA Hospital), to demonstrate a correlation between colonization of water sources with legionella and disease in veterans in several hospitals.[235]

Engineering controls must include the heating of tank-water to specific temperatures, administering proper chlorination, the redesigning of water pipes to prevent acute bends and stagnation, the regular changing of filters, and cleaning of humidifiers.

Contaminated Ice Machines

When I worked at the Wilmington VA hospital in Delaware, our laboratory found unusual bacteria called Mycobacterium gordonae in several sputum specimens. These organisms rarely cause true infections but can be confused with the bacteria which cause TB. Patients may receive unnecessary treatment. The late infection prevention nurse,

Elizabeth Fuhse RN, and I traced the source to dirty ice machines and water from the machines. Patients likely drank ice water contaminated with M. gordonae before submitting the sputum. Samples from surgical tissue, bone marrow or spinal fluid (all samples obtained with sterile technique) were never contaminated.[236] The ice machines were cleaned as per the manufacturers' recommendations. No patient was harmed, and none required treatment. But a clinician might have started treatment for TB mistaking the early report as consistent with tuberculosis. And there could have been an outbreak if the contamination was due to dangerous bacteria such as salmonella which can survive in ice for long periods.

Airborne Mold Infections

Construction poses special risks for patients whose immune systems are weakened by disease, chemotherapy and steroids. Dust often carries mold, especially aspergillus, which can be inhaled by susceptible patients. This is the same mold that caused the death of seven children in Seattle.[211, 212] Therefore, it is critical for hospitals and offices to seal off any areas under construction to minimize exposure to construction dust. Hospital can also install high efficiency particulate air filters in their operating and equipment storage rooms.

Marburg Virus infections

In 1967, seven of 31 laboratory workers in Marburg and Frankfurt in Germany and in Belgrade, Yugoslavia (now Serbia) died after developing fever, gastrointestinal symptoms, massive bleeding and shock. They had been doing experiments on African green monkeys imported from Uganda. This is how the Marburg virus, found in fruit bats in Africa, was first identified as a deadly disease. The patients had inhaled air contaminated with the virus.

Nowadays, patients with TB, chicken pox or dangerous airborne diseases are admitted to negative air pressure rooms which suck the air out and vent it to the atmosphere for rapid dilution. Thus "stale" contaminated air is not recirculated.

Hot tubs and whirlpools

Patients have developed bacterial skin infections such as pimples and pustules from bacteria (Pseudomonas aeruginosa) after exposure to whirlpools and spas which were not cleaned with diluted bleach regularly.

Flowers, fruit and raw vegetables

Hospitals request patients on chemotherapy not to have flowers in the room or to consume raw vegetables because they are commonly contaminated by bacteria and it is hard to disinfect such items.

***

PREVENTION OF OTHER CAUSES OF HARM

The journey to zero harm is incomplete if we fail to address risks other than hospital-acquired infections.

Poor communication

"The single biggest problem in communication is the illusion that it has taken place." Bernard Shaw is credited with this quotation, but it is more likely that these or similar words were used first by William H. Whyte, a journalist and a best-selling author, who wrote about organizations and public spaces. His instructional "Fortune" article was designed to encourage improved communication within the business domain. He wrote "The great enemy of communication, we find, is the illusion of it. We have talked enough; but we have not listened. And by not listening we have failed to concede the immense complexity of our society—and thus the great gaps between ourselves and those with whom we seek understanding."[237]

Patients are shocked to hear that most doctors work in isolation with few interactions with their colleagues or the team. The reliance of doctors on bloated chart notes with misleading cut and paste information, rather than direct conversations, is a dangerous trend and habit.

The journey to zero harm will fail unless we address this flaw in our system. It is the single most important cause of harm. A system which incorporates team meetings, multidisciplinary conferences, and timely consultations for complex illnesses and proper handoffs can go a long way to prevent harm. We have the technology and tools for communication including the humble telephone.

Transfers to long term care (LTC) Facilities

A transfer from a hospital to nursing home is one of the most dangerous times for the patient. In a study of 555 individuals who were followed for 45 days in 32 randomly selected facilities in six New England states, Kapoor et al found that adverse events developed in nearly four of ten discharges (40%) from the hospital back to LTC. They included pressure ulcers, skin tears, falls with injuries, infections and drug toxicity. Most were preventable or ameliorable. The events were deemed serious (38%), life-threatening (7.4%) and fatal (2.1%).[238] Hospitals could do a much better job communicating with LTC facilities.

Quality of nursing Homes or long-term care facilities (LTC)

The odor of urine or feces, when visiting a nursing home, is a warning sign. If patients appear unkempt, are strapped to chairs, have soiled clothing and sheets, or have food all over their bed, you know that the place is understaffed or uncaring. Most LTC facilities do not attract well-trained and highly motivated people because of low salaries, poor benefits and the need for physical strength and stamina. It is exhausting to look after feeble, elderly patients, especially those with dementia, who need help with feeding, bathing, ambulation and turning from side to side every two hours to prevent bedsores. The physical and emotional toll on health care workers leads to turnover, and occasional abuse of elderly or disabled residents. It is projected that 20% of the population will be over age 65 soon and that there will not be enough workers to care for them.

Patients have surprisingly little discretion on transfer from a hospital. They go where there is a timely bed. They may have more discretion changing NH to a more satisfying one once there. Nursing home care may cost $50- $100K each year, so it is wise to research where a hospital is planning to send your loved one and to check it out personally. Well-run nursing homes are clean, sunny, without odors, and are offer their residents' creature comforts, dignity, and respect.

Home health agencies

Home health care agencies face similar problems in recruiting. In 2014, when my mother needed a nursing aide daily for two hours, the agency sent a very pleasant young woman who had received no training. She did not know how to position a bench across the bathtub. I had to teach her.

Four years later, Asha, my terminally ill wife, needed palliative care under home hospice. We hired a company with an outstanding physician leader and administrative staff. An aide was assigned for 1.5 hours each day but rarely stayed more than 30 minutes claiming that was her lunch time, or that she had a back problem and was not supposed to bend. As days went by, she began to throw things in anger, refused to do certain chores and falsely claimed that the tasks were not part of her job description. My gentle wife, always pleasant and undemanding, pleaded with her but did not report this bad behavior to anyone fearing that the aide would get fired or that I would lose my temper. One day I caught the aide throwing a bucket on the floor with great force. The company was aware but had not intervened when other families had filed grievances. I spoke to the leaders and asked them to coach, retrain or fire her so she would not harm others.

Burdens on family members and caregivers

As described in an earlier chapter, the burden on caregivers is huge. My family and I, like millions of Americans, have cared for our loved ones with a sense of duty and gratitude. It is extremely difficult work. Family members mistakenly assume that such intense care and self-sacrifice will be needed for approximately 2 years. However, as two years pass, the realization comes that the period of caregiving will be longer and may stretch to five or more years.

Everyone is exhausted by this time. Full-time work becomes impossible, resulting in the loss of jobs or wages. Physical and emotional stress, as well as the loss of leisure time, breeds resentment and may result in elder abuse. Family squabbles arise when one sibling, often a female family member, must do a disproportionate amount of caregiving. It is a time when you discover who your real friends are.

Medicare will pay for respite care for exhausted caregivers for a few days each year. During this time, the patient is cared for in an inpatient hospice facility, thus allowing the caregiver to get some rest and even take a vacation. The burdens of elder care have been devastating. We need to find a better way to support caregivers.

Relatives are not compensated for the work they do. Caregiver exhaustion may lead to readmissions, higher costs, greater severity of illness and economic loss to society. If relatives are untrained, uninformed, not supported or reluctant, the patient is likely to be harmed.

Medications errors

Upon arrival in the ED, someone will ask for a list of current medications. Reliance on old records or memory is dangerous. The communication between the primary clinician and the hospital is extremely patchy or absent. Often a patient is too ill, confused or demented to provide a reliable history. Family members may not be available or may not know the details.

SICK AND SCARED

That is why I strongly recommend that each patient/family member keep a regularly updated smart phone app and/or a laminated list of meds with exact doses and frequency in their wallet or purse. A copy should be easily available at home in a medical folder. Each caregiver should have an updated copy. Old medication bottles and their contents should be disposed of according to local regulations. Hoarding them creates confusion and errors. I found it very useful to ask patients to haul in all their medications in a paper bag for me to inspect. This was particularly useful in an earlier HIV era when patients had to take a lot of pills each day. I rarely see physicians do that any longer.

The skill and insight of patients and families to understand and deal with diseases varies greatly. Ultimately, we will likely get much better results in safety by refining our processes and protocols than by trying to train an endless number of individual family members.

Polypharmacy

Patients in America get far too many pills. These are often "just in case" remedies for constipation, insomnia, agitation, mild pain, severe pain, breakthrough pain, and so on. All medications are potential poisons. That includes the over-the-counter medications which people pop every time a new symptom arises. That comment applies also to "natural" unregulated remedies.

Discharge medications

Discharge is a dangerous time for patients. Fairly well stabilized patients may see a whole new list of medications they were not aware they were getting. For example, new meds may be given for diabetes or hypertension and old ones discontinued without the patient's knowledge. Patients may begin to use the new and old ones at home simultaneously. A physician error may cause the patient to get a wrong drug or dose. It is always wise to check and confirm what has changed before discharge. Once you are out of the hospital, it will be nearly impossible for you to reach the doctor (hospitalist or resident) who discharged you.

One patient suffered disastrous consequences from internal bleeding when the physician mistakenly prescribed warfarin (Coumadin) a blood thinner, three times daily instead of once daily.

Some doctors dictate a discharge summary 1-2 days before the actual date of discharge as a favor to the colleagues who will see the patient later. This is common and extremely dangerous because meds may change in the last 48 hours of stay, or the clinical condition might change.

Look Alike and Sound Alike (LASA) drugs

Look alike and sound alike (LASA) drugs require special care. This is a common and hazardous risk of hospitalization. Hundreds of LASA drugs are included in the list prepared by the Institute for Safe Medication practices.[239] The key is constant vigilance. Look out for errors such as wrong patient name, wrong pill dose or wrong frequency.

Drug Costs

Physicians do not know the cost of most of the tests they order and the drugs they prescribe. They may be aware that patients have financial hardships but just do not know how to circumvent those difficulties. Physicians or other staff members can help patients obtain very expensive drugs by calling the manufacturer directly and pleading for help. In my experience, that has been effective almost every time, but it takes much time to make those contacts, get approvals and get the prescription filled. The pharmaceutical firms should be commended for supporting the needs of poor patients.

Additionally, I agree with the recommendation from the American College of Physicians that prescribers have an idea what it is going to cost the patient and to find cheaper but effective alternatives. If health care workers do not do so, it is more than likely that the patient will not fill that prescription or take lower doses than recommended.

SICK AND SCARED

Over the counter (OTC) drugs

I mentioned a patient who had kidney failure due to an OTC drug. Patients often assume these drugs must be safe because the FDA allows such sales, but many are dangerous, especially for the elderly. Among them are the anti-inflammatory agents such as aspirin, Motrin, ibuprofen, Aleve which can cause life threatening bleeding from the stomach and/or kidney failure. The first thing a kidney specialist looks for in patients with kidney failure is whether the patient has taken OTC pain relievers. It is reversible if identified quickly.

Acid in the stomach is nature's way of killing bacteria. Agents which reduce stomach acid (antacids such as Tums, Maalox, and numerous generics, histamine blockers such as Zantac, and proton pump inhibitors such as Nexium and others) can predispose to pneumonia and C diff. The proton pump inhibitors may also worsen osteoporosis. They should only be advised if the risk does not outweigh the benefits.

Falls

Falls are the leading cause of fatal and nonfatal injuries among adults aged ≥65 years (older adults). During 2014, approximately 27,000 older adults died because of falls; 2.8 million were treated in emergency departments for fall-related injuries, and approximately 800,000 of these patients were subsequently hospitalized. Bergen et al reported that 28.7% of those over the age 65 had fallen in 2014 (29 million people).[240] The crude mortality numbers from falls increased from 51.6 per 100,000 in 2000 to 122.2 per 100,000 in 2016, and so has the mortality. Mortality rates rise with age and are higher for men than they are for women.[241]

Age, infirmity, medication side effects, clutter in the room (such as cords and wires) and dim lighting create a risk for falls.

Hospitals try to stratify risk for patients and tag the charts of high-risk patients routinely. That risk score empowers staff to take precautions and to use bed alarm systems. Patients dislike the restrictions imposed by such devices and are annoyed by frequent false alarms. What they hate most is being escorted to the bathroom and the staff peering at their butt during what is supposed to be highly private ritual. It is an undignified intrusion into their privacy and sometimes culturally offensive. Nurses are, however, bound by safety rules and must escort the patient. Stepping away for a moment and hearing the awful thud of a patient falling is everyone's nightmare. It leads to reprimands for the nurse and accusations of negligence and litigation from the family.

Hospitals employ "sitters" for patients at risk. Nursing students or aides are paid a salary simply to sit at the bedside and are asked to keep an eye on patients at risk for falling. Does this strategy work? I remember sitting five feet from my wife when she misjudged where the chair was and hit the ground. There was a sickening sound of a broken bone. It happened so quickly that I could not have stopped the fall if I were Superman. The same thing happened again a year later. Except for yelling for help, sitters can do little to physically restrain a fall. A recent study suggests that we need to revisit this intervention because it may be ineffective and costly.[242]

Bed sores

Elderly, infirmed, exhausted, malnourished, or unconscious patients are at great risk for pressure ulcers. Patients who are not turned every two hours may suffer bed sores because the pressure cuts off the blood supply to the skin. The sore may get infected and burrow deeper into muscle and bone. Bacteria may enter the blood stream and cause shock and death. I have seen bed sores where the hole is deep, foul-smelling, where one can see the metal prosthesis inserted into the hip years ago. This is a nightmare situation for the patient. The wound requires debridement, packing, and/or plastic surgery to cover the hole with a muscle flap, antibiotics for weeks-on-end and arranging for expensive custom air mattresses.

The best protection is constant motion, repositioning every 2 hours, and immediate care of damaged skin. This is easier said than done. It requires physical strength to turn patients, especially if they are morbidly obese. Patients forget, or they are reluctant or too weak to change positions every few hours on their own. Paralyzed and sedated patients may feel no pain. Units which have zero bed sores are a testament to the tenacity and devotion of our nurses who may be the only ones who inspect the skin. Pressure sores are now a reportable event for hospitals and nursing homes.

Malnutrition

Patients often get malnourished in the hospital for a variety of reasons: they may have no appetite, are vomiting, nauseated or kept NPO (nothing by mouth) for a test or for surgery. Few patients enjoy hospital food, and some are repelled by the appearance or smell of hospital food. Most patients can handle withdrawal of nutrition for a few days but may need artificial nutrition later.

Artificial feeding involves the placement of a tube into the stomach either through the mouth or by an incision on the abdomen skin. Nutrients, supervised by trained dieticians, are provided through such tubes. There is also the option of intravenous nutrition by placing a catheter into the chest vein or neck. Both alimental feeding and intravenous feeding carries the risk of infections or surgical complications while placing the tubes. Malnourished patients do not heal well, need longer hospital stays and take much longer to recover their strength and energy levels.

Emotional harm

Patient grievances range from perceived rudeness, inefficiency, delays, huge bills, condescending or mean doctors and nurses, bad food, and a wrong diagnosis. I see these all complaints as opportunities to learn and improve. Others see it as a nuisance and send generic corporate letters which apologize for the patient's "inconvenience or experience" but do nothing to remedy the situation or to learn from it.

I have seen staff members scoff at complains about hospital bills even though we know they are often incorrect. The assumption that the patient wants to get out paying a bill is unfair. It is most irritating to have leaders say there is "no opportunity for improvement" and "close the case." Most patients do not pick up pen and paper to write letters to the CEO unless they are truly upset or feel humiliated. Dismissing their letters as unimportant is a disservice to the patient safety and satisfaction effort. The patient is the reason for our existence and to manage their concerns sincerely is our duty.

PART 9

TIPS FOR PATIENT SAFETY

Most people will need medical care sometime in their lifetime even if they follow all the recommendations for healthy living. They should know that the care they will receive will be excellent much of the time. However, there are significant risks to life and limb even in the finest hospitals in our nation. Here are 100 tips for patient safety and well-being.

Lifestyle changes

1. Stop smoking now. Each puff on the cigarette is shortening your life and will cause untold misery later. Some people quit "cold turkey." Others need help from a doctor. Keep trying until you succeed. E-cigarettes are not safe substitutes.
2. Secondhand smoke is deadly. Be a role model to your family and keep them safe.
3. Brush and floss your teeth at least once daily to prevent tooth decay, inflammation and heart disease.
4. Lose weight if you are overweight. Getting close to the ideal body weight -or just below it- may prevent hypertension, diabetes, heart disease, strokes and knee arthritis.
5. Weight loss is a matter of calories in (eat less) and calories out (exercise more).

6. Plant-based diets, with or without poultry, fish and an occasional steak are fine.
7. Stay hydrated. Avoid sugary sodas, salt, snacks and sweetened juices.
8. Enjoy a glass of red wine in the evening but excessive drinking, especially in smokers, correlates with cancers of the head and neck, fetal abnormalities.
9. Exercise can be going to a gym, doing yard work ("weeds are your friends!" according to my friend Dr. Joan DelFattore), walking, running, avoiding elevators.
10. Keep your mind active. Read, write, solve puzzles and think.
11. Listen to music. Tap your feet. Clap. Move. Dance.
12. Laugh a lot. Be silly.
13. Exit the rat race. No one wins. The rewards are fleeting. You have nothing to prove to others.
14. Find a few minutes of peace, quiet and solitude each day to reflect.
15. Try to learn something new every day.
16. Loneliness is an American epidemic today. Mingle with people.
17. Be curious. Keep learning. Attend lectures, musicals, plays and community events.
18. Volunteer. Help others. It gives you inner happiness and a purpose in life.
19. Avert Alzheimer's disease by being involved physically and mentally with others.
20. Age is just a number. Live your life with grace and gratitude. Avoid self-pity.

Preventive maintenance for you and your family

21. Find a good primary care clinician and see him/her at least once a year. The main purpose is to check weight, BP, catch

up on vaccinations, and check for hearing or visual problems, depression, dietary habits, personal wellness and fitness.

22. Doctors who are dually certified in integrative or Western medicine will give you the care you desire.
23. Do not judge your doctor by his/her dress, accent, appearance, skin color, gender, religion or national origin. You may miss out on a great doctor.
24. If you want 24/7 access and can afford it, go to a concierge or direct primary care doctor.
25. Experienced advanced practice nurses (nurse practitioners) will give you good primary care.
26. Bad vibes, lack of chemistry, rude staff, and inefficiency are reasons to switch doctors.
27. Buy a home blood pressure (BP) monitor. It could prevent a stroke, kidney disease, heart attacks and death.
28. Buy an inexpensive fingertip pulse oximeter to measure your oxygen levels if you have heart or lung disease or even as a signal to worry about COVID-19.
29. God and religion do not forbid vaccination. Urge your family and friends to accept vaccines.
30. It is best to get the flu shot 2-4 weeks before the flu season generally begins in your area. Vaccines given too early may wear off.
31. If you are sick, don't be a hero, and stay home.
32. Get routine cancer screening especially for breast and colon cancer.
33. Insist that everyone cleans their hands with alcohol or soap and water before touching you.
34. Avoid the ED for minor illness. You will irritate the staff, wait a long time and get a huge bill.
35. An urgent care center will serve you quickly and at lower cost for most common ailments.

36. Do not demand antibiotics for minor colds and coughs.
37. Learn how to read, write, and use a computer. It may be a matter of life and death.
38. Only 10% of patients check their online records. Get involved in your own care.
39. Google searches can be a double-edged sword. Use them as an adjunct for discussions with your doctor.
40. Don't have a car? Call Uber or Lyft both inexpensive options for local travel. You are worth it.
41. You have a right to get copies of your records, at a reasonable cost, and in a timely fashion.
42. Caring for a loved one and are exhausted? Ask for help from family, friends or respite programs.

Relationships with doctors and nurses

43. Treat your doctors and nurses as friends, confidants, and well-wishers. They care for you.
44. Let the doctor know you have many questions, ahead of time, so he/she can plan your visit.
45. Asking too many questions is safer than asking none.
46. A long wait in the office or ED means someone is sicker than you are. Don't curse the doctor.
47. A good doctor is always slower than the one who smiles, waves and disappears.
48. Send thank you notes to your doctor and nurse. They will never forget. It might even prompt them to do the same.
49. Some doctors and nurses say very little but care a lot. Empathy has many shapes.
50. Be good to nurses who do backbreaking work every day.
51. Be kind to staff. They may be depressed, exhausted, stressed or burnt out.

52. Do not tolerate rudeness from any staff member. Report them to patient relations staff.
53. Just because you don't like the diagnosis, it does not mean the doctor is wrong.
54. It is your right to get second opinions.
55. Don't knock doctors for their high salaries. They train for many years, work long hours and the job is emotionally draining and risky.
56. Ask the doctor how his/her day is going and about his family or vacation plans. You might spark some joy in someone.
57. Express grievances calmly to office staff. Seek an amicable resolution.
58. Writing bad online reviews anonymously is cowardly. Refrain from this.
59. If you wish to sue, be fair and ask your lawyer to exclude those who cared for you honestly.

Hospital Care

60. Check the Hospital Compare website at Medicare.gov for the quality of hospitals.
61. Do not go to your local hospital if it has a low rating or reputation. It is worth traveling further.
62. Hospitals have the best staffing from 8 AM to 4 PM Monday through Friday.
63. Avoid weekends and nights for admissions unless it is an emergency. Mortality rates are higher.
64. Choose a Monday or Tuesday for elective admissions, tests or procedures. You will be safer.
65. Carry an updated summary of your medical problems, operations, allergies and medications.

66. Ask what "observation status" means before signing. It may help you avoid bankruptcy.
67. Ask why tests are being done. Insist on getting results and explanations.
68. Ask staff to weigh you (*no guesses*) because drug doses depend upon actual weight.
69. Ask the discharge planner nicely at discharge if future appointments could be made for you.
70. Most patients forget verbal instructions quickly. Ask for permission to record or take notes.
71. Never leave your cognitively impaired loved one alone in the hospital at any time.
72. Patients who are not impaired will also be safer if a family member/friend is around.
73. Make sure the nurse has direct phone numbers for family members or close friends.
74. Make sure the staff knows about your wishes about intensive care and resuscitation.
75. Have documents such as a living will, power of attorney and a list of your doctors handy.
76. Do not torture your loved one if their time has come. Let them go with dignity.
77. You may see a different "covering" doctor each day or week. Ask for a business card/name.
78. You have the right to choose a specialist/consultant when one is needed.
79. Ask consultants and physiotherapists if they need to visit daily. You are paying for each visit.
80. Ask the surgeon how much experience he has with the procedure to be done.

81. Ask who will do the actual operation. Some surgeons go from room to room supervising multiple operations. This is known as "concurrent surgery," and it is frowned upon.
82. Do not sign consent forms without a satisfactory explanation of potential complications.
83. If you have physician friend, ask him/her to "keep an eye" on your loved one.
84. Make sure the call button, food tray and glass of water are within reach.
85. Never use family/friends as interpreters. Use official medical interpreters.
86. Call an RRT if you feel your loved one is worse, and the staff is not addressing your concerns.
87. Wear non-slip socks, have beds lowered and the side rails up. Remove clutter.
88. When in the hospital, or even at home, keep the head of the bed up at about 30 degrees to prevent aspiration pneumonia.
89. Take your time before standing up; don't walk if you are feeling dizzy or light-headed.

Medications

90. Buy generic drugs from big box pharmacies (cheaper) rather than smaller pharmacies. The cost difference between brand names at pharmacies is not significantly different.[243] It is also worth checking out https://www.goodrx.com/ to find discounts on your prescription if you are paying out of pocket. You cannot use those coupons if insurance covers your prescriptions.
91. Wrist bands, allergy labels and questions about your ID are safety measures. Don't get irritated.
92. Know the names of each medicine you take (instead of the "blue, little, bitter or round" pill)

93. Some doctors prefer to see all your pill bottles. Bring them to each visit.
94. Ask to use your own home medications when admitted. You will save money.
95. Ask why any pill or injection is being given.
96. Don't distract nurses who are preparing meds. That leads to errors.
97. Check your prescriptions upon discharge from the hospital to make sure they are accurate.
98. Check medications you get from your local pharmacy. Pharmacists in retail pharmacies are struggling with their workload -prescriptions, phone calls, giving flu shots, counseling patients, calling doctors and insurance companies- while trying to satisfy their employer's performance standards for productivity. Errors are common and dangerous.

Bills

99. Most hospital bills are inaccurate. Be careful before paying up.[48] Ask for an itemized bill. You may see many surprise items. Self-pay (uninsured) patients pay far more than the insured. Negotiate for a substantial (30-50%) discount and a reasonable payment plan.
100. Report fraud by the clinic, hospital or doctor to insurance or Medicare.

PART 10

TIPS FOR PHYSICIAN SUCCESS AND WELLNESS

Why did we choose this profession?

Andre Machado of the Cleveland Clinic's Neurologic Institute reminds physicians:

"Remember why we went into healthcare. Healthcare is changing rapidly and will continue to change. The demands on physicians and all healthcare professionals are greater and will continue to evolve. Burnout is now part of the vocabulary across all organizations and it is sometimes quite visible. We all went into health care for a reason, a calling. When constantly stressed and rushed, we can lose that perspective, that memory. I hope that each of us can start the day reminding ourselves why is it that we do what we do and how much our patients rely on us to mitigate their pain, their suffering, their anxiety. By keeping that perspective constant — while acknowledging the pressures— we will do well for our patients and their experience with healthcare...."[244]

We have a responsibility to protect our patients, to look after each other and to advocate for change at the national level. Here are 66 tips for physician wellbeing.

1. Live neither in the past nor in the future, but let each day absorb all your interest, energy and enthusiasm. The best preparation for tomorrow is to live today superbly well. [245]

2. The practice of medicine will be very much as you make it - to one a worry, a care, a perpetual annoyance; to another, a daily job and a life of as much happiness and usefulness as can well fall to the lot of man, because it is a life of self-sacrifice and of countless opportunities to comfort and help the weak-hearted, and to raise up those that fall. [246]

3. The clinician who keeps an eye on the watch while in the wards is rarely successful. [247]

4. Listen to your patient, he/she is telling you the diagnosis.[248]

5. No man is happy or safe without a hobby.[249]

6. Life-long learning is essential.[250]

7. Plan your day the night before. Do each task calmly.

8. Always be kind to all patients. They come to you seeking help.

9. Do not interrupt the patient because you are in a hurry.

10. Consider the patient's personal, social and financial circumstances when planning treatment.

11. Admit mistakes quickly. You will sleep better.

12. Respect each patient regardless of his/her social status.

13. Do not abandon your patients in the twilight of their life.

14. Don't tower over your patients or look down at them. They are already scared. Sit at eye level.

15. Listen to their amazing stories.

16. Support them with kind gestures; a smile, a touch, a nod.

17. Encourage patients to ask questions.

18. Be patient. Do not rush them out. Give them the time their care requires.

19. If your patient repeatedly rejects sound advice, it is reasonable to ask the person politely to find another doctor. This is particularly true when parents continue to deny their children necessary vaccines.[251]

20. If several patients write scathing online reviews, try to understand why they are so upset.
21. If you are sued and you are sure you did nothing wrong, stand your ground.
22. It is reasonable to counter-sue a patient who files an obviously frivolous lawsuit against you.
23. If a patient wants to leave your practice, help the person with the transfer of records. Don't take it personally.
24. If I cannot do great things, I can do small things in a great way. Martin Luther King Jr.[252] Say something nice to each patient
25. Always be professional with colleagues, staff and patients.
26. Do not bad-mouth other doctors. It is not useful. They will retaliate.
27. Do not be arrogant. Peter Pronovost said, "Medicine operates like a private club of self-styled deities where the entrance requirement is an MD." [253, 254] Humility is a great virtue. Flaunting one's financial or educational status diminishes the respect others have for you.
28. Go out of your way to help someone. A doctor and nurse, during a lull in the ED schedule, found the time to talk to and help a homeless man. The nurse cleaned his face and combed his hair. The team gave him food, arranged transportation and found a shelter. On a busy day, he would have been just discharged out on the street. The anonymous author speaks of our profession and its humanity and how we can reach out to even the most disenfranchised people on the planet.[255]
29. Take it easy. Slow down. Take a break. A moment for reflection makes the next task easier.
30. Bite your tongue before you say something which will hurt someone. Or walk away.
31. Control your temper. Thumping the desk or mumbling profanities never helps.

32. Do not make promises to patients or family that you might be unable to keep.
33. Do not judge others unless you are flawless.
34. Pharmaceutical sales representatives are professionals who have a job to do. Don't insult them by asking them to bring pizza or dinner as a condition for meeting them. You can afford to buy your own.
35. When was the last time you thanked the environmental service staff for cleaning your office? They work hard too.
36. Do not humiliate people who do not rise to your standards. People are not all equally capable.
37. Be humble and listen to others respectfully.
38. Stop whining. It is irritating.
39. Do not take short cuts. It might kill someone.
40. Do not ever do unnecessary procedures to line your own pockets or overcharge patients. Resist temptation.
41. Make each one of your notes meaningful.
42. Don't click on templates thoughtlessly. It will bring in money but bother your conscience.
43. Do not plagiarize notes written by others. However, if the patient is unable to provide a history, it is OK to state that the history is based on a review of notes by other physicians.
44. Don't use offensive terms to describe patients in the chart. It is not right. Moreover, patients can read their chart notes.
45. Laugh heartily each day.
46. Good work takes time. Be methodical with each task before moving on to the next one.
47. Multi-tasking is a myth. So, don't aspire to it. It only breeds carelessness.

48. Stop bashing outside agencies which oversee safety and quality. The Joint Commission and the CMS hold us accountable and have catalyzed the journey to zero harm.
49. Be polite and respectful when nurses call for help. They are amazing partners.
50. Call consultants directly if you are asking for an urgent consultation. It is good manners, establishes good relationships and saves the consultant much time.
51. Ask for multidisciplinary meetings for your complicated patients.
52. Leave the profession or find nonclinical work if you begin to dislike patients or clinical work.
53. On call nights or weekends, just assume you will be extremely busy and tackle each task methodically. If you are overwhelmed, call your partners to help. It is a safety measure.
54. If you see a colleague in distress, do not walk away. Reach out and offer to help.
55. Spend some time with colleagues in the lounge and ask about their work and families.
56. If you are fed up with conventional jobs in offices and hospitals, consider work as a locum tenens physician. These short contracts- typically for weeks or months- pay well, cover the costs of travel, meals, lodging and transportation, zero overhead, no night calls and no long-term commitment.
57. If oppressed by work conditions and nearing burnout, do not withdraw into a shell. Seek help from friends and family or senior colleagues. Hospitals have contracts with outside agencies where you can get confidential help.
58. Do not withdraw from life. Loneliness is a deadly scourge and a national epidemic. Find your tribe.
59. Encourage your children to become health care professionals. The rewards are worth the sacrifices.

60. Be constructive, honest and open. Health care has its share of hypocrites and sycophants.
61. Participate on committees. Seek a dialogue with leaders when you have a idea for improvement.
62. Partner with like-minded colleagues to improve things.
63. Become a meaningful participant in your professional organizations on behalf of our patients and colleagues.
64. Ours is a noble profession. Keep it noble.
65. Fight tooth and nail for your patients. You can make a difference in their lives.
66. Support electoral candidates who are committed to health care reforms.

PART 11

THE SEVEN PILLARS OF HEALTHCARE REFORM

The White House is red, but some states are blue;
So, health policy by litigation, is all that we do.

~Meril Pothen[256]

The path to reform is fraught with extraordinary difficulties. Small incremental changes will not suffice. Americans want high-quality health care at an affordable cost but feel our leaders are not listening. It is time to demand change.

Several friends whom I respect greatly have lauded my enthusiasm for health care reform but feel that it is simply a wish list with no realistic chance of success. They cite the difficulties in overcoming resistance from powerful vested interests. While discouraging, cynicism cannot be the way forward. I refuse to accept the idea that this nation does not have the desire, the will or the intelligence to find a solution.

A major problem is that most leaders have taken strong entrenched positions from which they cannot easily extricate themselves. With goodwill, civility and brainstorming, we can create a model which others might envy. Most countries which now have universal health care did not have it at one time. What was their journey to reform like? What led them to the models they now have? How did they get the consensus to move forward?

Dr. Brad Spellberg's recent book *Broken, Bankrupt and Dying*[257] is one of the most comprehensive accounts of how other nations have designed successful systems from scratch. The author is an outstanding scientist and thought leader who says that there are enough models to suit different ideologies. They range from government ownership of the entire system to a private-public partnership. He has carefully analyzed the implications of imitating systems such as the ones in Europe, Australia and New Zealand.

A striking conclusion is that the implementation of universal coverage and a single payer system would lower costs for individuals, businesses and save money for the nation while providing excellent care. He describes how a reform plan in California failed because of misinformation in the press about the costs. If they had implemented that plan, the state, which has one of the world's largest economies, would have saved more than $35 billion annually while providing health care to everyone. It is unnecessary, he says, to antagonize insurers, pharmaceutical companies and hospitals. Universal policies could include an option to buy supplemental policies akin to the Fast Trac, EZ Pass on expressways or Medicare Advantage plans. Hospitals do not have to be owned by the government. Health systems in Canada, Australia, New Zealand and other countries work in collaboration with private hospitals and clinicians. Israel has five private insurers whose fiscal conduct is carefully monitored.

The US has a loose patchwork of "fee-for-service" systems for different populations all with their own rules and oversight structure. For example, there is the state-controlled Medicaid program for the poor, and a federally supported Medicare program for the elderly and those with end stage kidney disease. We have the federally supported VA system for veterans who must satisfy complex eligibility rules. And a health care system exists for active military personnel. However, all other groups are either dependent on employment or cannot afford insurance even though they work hard.

Countries with successful health care systems have several things in common. Everyone is assured basic medical care. Everyone pitches in with a payroll tax. Employers are not burdened with insurance costs. Private supplemental insurance is available for those who want it and can afford it. The salary gap between surgeons, specialists and primary care clinicians is narrower. Most have a single payer system whether their doctors and hospitals are private or publicly owned. Their national health care plans are driven by fairness and compassion rather than ideology. And their citizens are healthier than Americans.

We too can build a win-win system for all without dragging in ideology or partisan politics.

What are the obstacles in the US?

Patients and their doctors want change but feel helpless. Medical organizations cannot alienate their physician members, especially the high earning specialists. Primary care specialties will demand more. Surgeons will not accept less. Most doctors will not join a national union to force change. And if they do, they will not take any collective action which may harm their patients. We have been brainwashed into believing that a strike by doctors is unethical. Thus, we have lost our voice.

Insurers depend on controlling costs. They have several techniques such as paying providers less, restricting access to care or allowing pharmaceutical manufacturers to compete on price when they offer competing products. Pharmaceutical firms and device makers will fight any plan to curb costs and profits tooth and nail. They have responsibilities to their shareholders. Current politicians, acutely aware of the hardships people face, will not be agents of change. They are beholden to vested interests whose main goal is wealth, not health. The 4,000 lobbyists for industry outnumber 535 members of Congress by a ratio of 8:1. Thirty nine of the forty members who serve on health and finance committees benefit from corporate largesse.

Critics have clouded the debate by pitting the choices as an ideologic battle between capitalism and socialism rather than taking the middle ground and asking, "What is good for our people, our economy and our nation?"

Even so, I am cautiously optimistic that change is around the corner. There are several reasons for the sunny outlook.

1. The COVID-19 pandemic is proof that our health care structure is sick, and many of our politicians are out of their depth in matters of science and epidemiology. Americans have paid an extremely heavy price for this unforgivable failure of leadership. People will vote for change.

2. In January 2020, before the COVID-10 pandemic hit us, Americans listed health care as extremely important (35%) followed by terrorism (34%), guns (34%) education (33%) immigration (28%) and climate change (26%). When the categories "extremely important and very important" are combined, the polls show that the economy (84%) is the top concern, followed by education (83%), health care (81%) terrorism (80%), immigration (74%) and climate change (55%).[258]

3. Americans desperately seek and need a simpler and better health system.

4. Young Americans are more liberal, less driven by ideology and support universal health care. Charlotte Alter, a well-known Time Magazine journalist, in her just-published book *The Ones We've Been Waiting For: How a new generation of leaders will transform America* argues that young people will vote for health care as a basic human right.[259]

5. The risks health care workers took to save lives during this pandemic has bridged a chasm. Patients and physicians are now allies in the same battle.

6. We know we need Disruptive Innovation — as the late Clayton Christensen would say — but not by moving doctors around, but rather by redefining the goals of health care, to shift from an emphasis on acute care to prevention and wellness. The current model should be "broken up, redefined and repurposed."[125,126] The four main principles of Disruptive

Innovation are summarized in a Harvard Business Review article. Basically, an established business successfully takes care of core customers. A new entrant disrupts the dominance of the incumbent business which has not catered to the needs of all customers by introducing a new concept or service. The idea becomes popular and the new entrant then attracts core customers from the established business. The new entrant fills a niche, lowers cost and then takes over the original business. At this point disruption has occurred.[260]

7. For the first time in its 105 year history, the American College of Physicians, with a membership of over 165,000 doctors, has supported universal coverage and a single payer system.

8. My friend Dr. Richard Plotzker wrote: "All of the countries that have national health insurance at one time didn't. How they got from not having it to finding it indispensable is one of those lessons of history that have a lot of potential but never seem to be part of any American plan to go from nothing to something." (Personal Communication, August 20, 2020)

It is time for people to express what they need and deserve. The old guard must go and be replaced. Margaret Mead said, *"Never doubt that a small group of thoughtful, committed citizens can change the world; indeed, it's the only thing that ever has."* Do we dare to believe that this "small group" will be enlightened and compassionate politicians, corporate leaders, patient advisors and physicians?

1st Pillar: The Political Imperative

Harry Truman was thwarted by the AMA from going further with his health reform agenda. Lyndon Johnson got the biggest reforms: Medicare and Medicaid. While the protections were for a defined subset of the population, they were comprehensive and are so ingrained that nobody would undermine them now. Bill Clinton failed in his efforts to reform health care because of fierce opposition from vested interests including the AMA. President Obama's Patient Protection and Affordable Care Act (known as ACA) became law in March 2010 because he was willing to compromise, had a supermajority of votes in the Senate and knew that he would not get everything he wanted. His pragmatic approach to accept something less than perfect got bipartisan support. Indeed, the insurance companies would never have agreed to the ACA but for the billions of dollars given to them to "subsidize" lower premiums. The ACA gave health care access to 20 million of the 50 million uninsured. However, the ACA did not hurt corporate profits at all. Politicians protected their benefactors. It was an imperfect bill but better than what we had before.

If voters truly want a universal health care system with a single payer, lower costs, and higher quality, they must vote for candidates who want the same. They would speak for us regardless of their party affiliation. Their tasks would be the following:

1. The creation of a universal health care system for all which would be funded by a universal tax on individuals. It could be Medicare for all, or it could be a Medicare-like plan for those who want other options, including private insurers. (The ACP has advocated such plans recently).
2. The elimination of employer costs for health care, thus saving $20,000 per employee
3. The institution of nominal co-pays, coinsurance, and deductibles. A wise colleague, Dr. Richard Plotzker, quips "if you pay nothing, it is worth nothing." That is why insurers insist on co-pays, even if nominal, and write it into their provider contracts. Even Medicaid and some VA services have started instituting co-pays.
4. The inclusion of dental and eye coverage.
5. The elimination of "in network" plans.
6. Allowing the choice of affordable plans whether government, private or a combination with fixed prices. An example would be Israel's successful system which created an oligopoly where the five authorized companies can make money if they don't "misbehave." Each beneficiary selects a plan, or if they neglect

to select, they are assigned one for that year. The plans have a fixed price and compete for patients with what they offer for that price, regulated by mandated services. They do have networks within the authorized plan, but anyone can change plans at the next open season. (Personal Communication, Dr. Richard Plotzker, Email August 20, 2020)

7. To permit competition for mandated services and regulations to prevent abuse by insurers.
8. To ensure the right to choose any physician and the right to a hospital of choice.
9. To create a standardized list of prices for supplies, services, and surgery.
10. To create a system to identify fraud quickly.
11. To review the operations of "non-profit" institutions: their overheads and C-suite bloat.
12. Institute free medical school education -or debt forgiveness- for clinicians in return for service contracts and paybacks post-graduation.
13. To grant permanent residency to physicians with H1-B visas. (They have waited long enough).
14. To continue the requirement for quality improvement and harm reduction initiatives and penalties for failures to keep patients safe.
15. To extend the Sunshine Act for politicians who would be required to report any gift over $10 (just as doctors do) and prohibit legislators from serving on committees when they have a conflict of interest.

2nd Pillar: Treat patients as VIPs

The business of medicine must return to its roots. There is nothing more exhilarating than healing the bodies and minds of the wounded. We must make the patient care experience warm and pleasant.

Maya Angelou said, "I've learned that people will forget what you said, people will forget what you did, but people will never forget how you made them feel."

It is that simple. Take care of those who come to you! Make their lives easier. Give them the courtesy you would want for yourself. Put yourself in their shoes. We can start with basic manners, efficiency and anticipation of needs.

Easy appointments and check in:

Office schedules are inconvenient for working people. We can begin with online appointments, evening and weekend hours, courteous receptionists and automatic reminders. Patients are overwhelmed and may get lost in a hospital. Way-finding apps or maps, or even escorts, can be extremely helpful. Institute simple check-in systems, such as the ones being used at the University of Pittsburgh Medical Center, may help. They have recorded 600,000 fingerprints for a quick check in. Retinal scans might be the next technologic step. Singapore is now using facial recognition for various services.

Missed appointments:

No-show rates as high as 30-50% are a drain on clinic and hospital resources, revenue, and they are associated with worse clinical outcomes. Socioeconomic determinants of health -poverty, old age, cognitive decline, acute illness or lack of transportation- are serious problems which require special attention. Offering transportation to such patients is an inexpensive win-win strategy. It costs as little as $4 per ride for a visit easily recouped by the revenue generated by the visit and the wellness which accrues. Florida Blue announced on Nov 4, 2019 that it will be offering its million plus ACA Exchange Plan members transportation to clinic visits through a partnership with Lyft in the "Better You Strides Rewards Program" beginning in 2020. As a bonus, it will reduce pressures on parking spaces in hospitals.

SICK AND SCARED

Some procedures require that the patient be observed for a few hours before discharge. In a nation where so many are lonely, disabled or who live alone, we will need to make a provision to provide paid or volunteer force to help.

Home visits:

Dr, Jeffrey Benner, from Camden, New Jersey, noticed that a few patients from certain areas utilized medical services at a much higher rate that others in the area. Five percent of all patients accounted for 50% of annual health care spending and 1% accounted for 25% of the spending. He figured that focusing on these super-utilizers might improve their health and lower costs. Benner's idea of super-utilizers in hot spots led to the creation of the Camden Coalition of Healthcare providers. Atul Gawande describes how Dr. Benner and Dr. Rushika Fernadopoulle in Atlantic City have focused on the care of such high-risk populations with excellent results. Of course, keeping people healthy is "bad" for hospitals, emergency departments and pharmacies.[261]

It is known that approximately twenty percent of all discharged patients will be readmitted within 30 days. CMS has penalties for hospitals which exceed this number. Besides the penalty, it makes sense to identify such super-utilizers and manage them preemptively.

Careful follow up of discharged patients has been shown to be cost-effective. A review of transitional services in patients older than 75 who were discharged after treatment of heart failure showed that home nursing services were economically cost-effective compared to nurse case management or disease management clinics.[262] However, a study from Camden, NJ showed that readmission rates were identical (around 62%) for 800 super-utilizers randomized to get either usual care versus use of the Coalition's transition care program.[263]

We need to understand how the model should be tweaked to get better outcomes. The basic premise of keeping these patients well in their homes is still a good idea. Perhaps telemedicine, which has skyrocketed during the COVID-19 era, will be a potential solution. Patients could be examined remotely with sophisticated tools without touching them. Patients will find it very convenient.

Hospitality Business:

Hospitals must learn how top hotels get their reputation. The fountains, flowers and gardens are not a waste of resources. Children heal better when they are housed in cheerful rooms with bright colors which exude sunshine. Adults are no different. A nice, clean hospital with happy workers who truly love their job begins the healing process even before any medicine has been delivered. Patients do not fall as often when rooms are uncluttered. Hospitals should aspire for challenging benchmarks.

Safety:

This must be the paramount goal of all health care policies.

3rd Pillar: Give Clinicians "The Gift of Time"

Dr. Eric Topol, director and founder of the Scripps Research Translational Institute says we must give physicians and patients "the gift of time" and get back to where medicine was decades ago, when the relationship was characterized by a deep bond with trust and empathy. While doing research for the British National Health Service, a team of health care economists working with him calculated that "eliminating just one minute of keyboard entry time for doctors represented the equivalent of 400,000 hours of consultation time, or 230 full time physicians."[15] Clinician burnout is strongly related to the stress of trying to do important and necessary work in an incredibly short span of time. This time pressure inevitably leads to short cuts, stress and guilt. Institutions will never solve the problem of burnout unless they find ways to reduce physician burdens, increase visit times and take away tasks which do not require a medical degree. I believe this is the single most important priority to restore the patient physician relationship to what it used to be.

A single billing system would free doctors from the paperwork for numerous insurers given that almost half the visit time is currently spent on EMR work.[168]

Scribes:

Strategies to reduce burdens include the implementation of scribes who document histories, physical examination findings, presumed diagnosis and the management plan while the MD does her work. The efficiency of this system was evident to me during a visit to my eye doctor. During the 15-minute visit, she did not write a single note or click a single key. A signed note, with pictures of my retina, was handed to me at check out. The visit was perfect, professional and courteous.

According to Dr. Vishal Patel, a senior research investigator at the Value Institute at the Christiana Care and a Med/Peds faculty member, medical scribes are paid salaries in the $25,000 to $40,000 range. Scheduling two or more patients per day pays for the scribe. Other benefits include more timely and accurate documentation and less "pajama time" for the clinician. (Personal Communication, November 11th, 2019)

Voice to Text:

One could dictate a note while examining the patient. This tends to be a bit distracting for patients but has the advantage of saving time and informing the patient what the note will state. Improved dictation systems recognize different accents and create voice to type transcripts instantly.

Scribble:

Scribble replaces a live scribe. An individual, perhaps on another continent, listens remotely and types and submits a report within hours. This reduces physician EMR time by about 60%, saving 1-2 precious hours each day. Patient experience scores have improved where such systems have been used.[264]

Suki:

Google's voice-enabled digital assistant Suki can reduce the time needed to document a visit from 13 minutes to 3 minutes. The saved minutes are spent counseling, coaching, and providing direct care unencumbered by a computer screen. I see a future where robots gather the history, enter the symptoms into a search engine and produce a differential diagnosis, and the physician spends the rest of the time deciding the next steps with the patient.

4th Pillar: A Patient-Clinician Alliance

Christine Bechtel, a patient advocate and champion of consumer rights, writes "As a patient, I never understood the heartbreakingly human toll our system takes on clinicians." Adding, "Namely, I had no idea what working in this system was doing to you, our frontline clinicians-the humans we rely on for medical wisdom. Doctors, physician assistants, nurses, nurse practitioners, medical assistants, everyone......But now I see that when it feels like patients and clinicians are adversaries rather than allies, it's because the way the health care system is organized and financed is actually inhumane."

She calls for reengineering these relationships and for physicians to "reveal their authentic selves" by talking to patients about their suffering, adding" no one cares about your joy. They care about your pain."[265]

Clinicians and patients must push for national health care reform together. We are partners who want the same thing. This is the right time. Our elected leaders would be wise to heed the pleas of voters.

SICK AND SCARED

5th Pillar: Shift focus from acute care to preventive care

Imagine a large pothole on a busy commercial highway. It has resulted in numerous accidents, injuries and deaths. They build a major trauma center nearby to manage the injuries. It has attracted great talent and has gained a national reputation for miraculously saving lives which would otherwise have been lost for sure. In high demand, those who fix fractured skulls and broken bodies are coveted and command high salaries. A business of this size needs administrators by the truckload.

The poor residents of the neighborhood wonder why they didn't fix the pothole in the first place.

That hole in America is the lack of consistently good primary and preventive care. Primary care clinicians are not valued enough. The ones who wield a scalpel do fix the injury but do little to prevent it. Poor access to primary care is driving people into urgent care centers and emergency departments. If all citizens were to receive decent primary care in their own neighborhoods, there would be less pressure on emergency departments which "feed" hospital beds.

We pay lip service to the benefits of education, balanced diets, regular exercise, blood pressure checks, and prevention of obesity, diabetes, smoking cessation, drug abuse, safe housing, crime, social services, mental health, suicides, depression, loneliness, poverty, joblessness, homelessness and illiteracy. I have seen estimates of 24 to 42 million citizens who have no access to broadband internet. More than 36 million Americans cannot read. A majority is unable to identify countries on a world map or cities within the US. Thus, they will not be part of the technology revolution that is coming. We will need to find ways to reach them through community outreach, places of worship and public libraries.

Primary care must have a much bigger impact on society than fixing the damage caused by preventable diseases. Whether staffed by doctors, APNs or PA s, addressing the basic drivers of poor health will have a much greater impact in the future than all the shiniest hospitals we can build. We must make primary care attractive once again. I believe that clinicians with different types of training will come together, call a truce and find ways to align each other's skills for the benefit of patients.

6th Pillar: Administrative Reforms

Health care spending has hit the $3 trillion mark or $11,172 per person. Senator Elizabeth Warren, a proponent of Medicare for All, expects the costs to escalate to 11 trillion in a decade if we do nothing. That is simply unaffordable. We must cut costs. This battle cannot be won without legislation. Reforms at the national level have been discussed under pillar #1.

There is no need to reinvent the wheel each time. A single payer system and universal health care will immediately bring down administrative costs close to below 3% that Medicare spends compared to the 10-20% costs for private insurance. Additionally, the suffering of patients would be alleviated once private insurance denials for care are forbidden.

Courtesy:

Train the staff to be courteous, to go the extra mile and monitor their performance.

Access and abuse:

My friends tell me they are transferred from person to person, sometimes experience extremely arrogant and rude receptionists, and endure long delays and roadblocks when they seek appointments or copies of records.

SICK AND SCARED

Institutional humility

Institutional humility is a good thing. It is fine to brag about awards and recognition, but it is also important to acknowledge what is done badly, to apologize to patients and learn from mistakes.

Eliminate waste:

The elimination of waste includes the reduction of administrative staff, exorbitant salaries and other steps as outlined by Brent and Savitz at Intermountain Health.[266] Figure out the layers of processes which cost money at each step. Simplify. A daily blood count or a daily chest x-ray in the ICU wastes a lot of time and money without benefit. We need to practice with logic and commonsense.

Salaries:

Reduce salary disparities between primary care and specialists. Yes, there is the issue of supply and demand, to be sure. But a new surgical attending or specialist should not earn three times what an internist earns after three decades of flawless service.

Levels of authority:

The titles one sees in hospital administration would astound anyone who retired a decade ago. There are leaders for transformation, innovation, government affairs, consumerism, environment, diversity, talent retention, safety, quality, external affairs, finance, human resources, wellness, legal affairs, medical affairs, academic affairs, professionalism, peer review, graduate education, research, department chairs, vice chairs, assistants to the chair and vice chair, directors of this and that, several chiefs and chief medical officers, special advisors. And the list goes on. The hierarchy, and authority is often unclear, and everyone plays safe to be on the good side of bosses. I am sure there is room for streamlining, consolidation and work sharing in all these administrative jobs. Very few of them see patients or bring in revenue. Their salaries are generally rather generous compared to those in the trenches (and certainly for the hours worked).

Fewer hospitals and hospital beds:

As health care strategies change -to keep people well and prevent acute illness- we will need fewer acute care beds. Competition and rising costs have already driven many smaller and inefficient hospitals into bankruptcy and closure. This is particularly true for inner city and rural hospitals whose operating margins are much thinner than non safety-net hospitals. Consolidation of services into large high-quality medical centers is supposed to streamline operations and lower costs, but data suggest that such mergers raise costs and lower quality. We must try to understand why that should be.

Choose Wisely:

Choosing Wisely is an evidence-based program to ensure the judicious use of antibiotics and other resources, [111] but most institutions continue to do business as usual. It is often an un-enforced policy on paper. There ought to be restrictions on very expensive tests and procedures if a simpler test is as accurate and just as good. For example, a dialogue with a radiologist might reveal the best test for a certain diagnosis. This becomes an educational experience, and the patient gets the benefit of the institution's collective wisdom. Every clinician should not be permitted to order any test they want without some filters about appropriateness and cost effectiveness.

Fair Bills:

Fees schedules should be easily available. Bills should be itemized, accurate and comprehensible to lay people. A patient should be able to compare and shop around for services.

7th Pillar: Wise use of Technology

Technology offers many opportunities for increasing efficiency, creature comforts, and the gift of time for doctors, as well as improving our diagnostic abilities, and the ability to accomplish our tedious chores. Machines can take better histories, and they are more accurate than humans in diagnostics. Algorithms could lead to rapid diagnosis.

Machines can work 24/7, need no vacations or health benefits, and do not complain. Improved wearable technologies are new frontiers which offer exciting possibilities in diagnostics and epidemiology. In the words of Kevin Kelly,

"*Robots are here to stay. It is inevitable.*" They will make our lives better and our relationships stronger.

But we must never forget that the suffering of the sick and scared will always require the human touch.

PART 12

HOW SERVANT LEADERS ARE MAKING A DIFFERENCE IN A BROKEN HEALTHCARE SYSTEM

> *Gentlemen, I have a confession to make. Half of what we have taught you is in error, and furthermore we cannot tell you which half it is.*
>
> ~William Osler

There is a battle going on in hospitals across the nation, but this fight has no winners. The combatants are administrators who are pitted against doctors "in the trenches." The former, tired of hearing the moans and groans of the foot soldiers, hide in their badge-entry-only "fortresses," while the troops, ignored and powerless, seethe helplessly as they sink deeper into the abyss of cynicism and burnout.

This popular analogy to war is unfortunate because both groups share identical goals to take care of sick people with compassion while assuring quality, safety and financial stability. However, the two sides do not communicate well, little gets resolved and the cold war goes on.

Hospitals are now essentially run by an enlarging group of administrators who enact rules, regulations and edicts and displace hapless physicians who were once the captains of the ship but now have neither autonomy nor clout. Medical societies remained silent while administrative reforms were in process.

Most Chief Executive Officers (CEOs) start out with great intentions, but once the excitement abates, they begin to isolate themselves and suffer burnout just as physicians do. An average CEOs tenure is just under 10 years. In the first few years, they often dismantle everything their predecessor did (good and bad) to put their own brand on things. Leaders with too many priorities, land up achieving very few goals. In the latter part, they go with the flow and get more detached. The fire ebbs. There are other people eyeing the throne, in order to find the opportunities to advance their own brand, get name recognition...and the cycle goes on.

Physician burnout occurs when the physician feels neglected, excluded, voiceless and devalued by leadership. CEOs often surround themselves within a cocoon of compliant lieutenants. This would be fine if the deputies were fearless in speaking up. Generally, the outspoken ones get booted out. The sycophants shield the boss from the dissonance.

Great institutions are created by leaders who instill confidence and pride in their systems. What are the attributes of such good leaders? How does he/she create a milieu where individuals feel valued and heard within a culture of gentle togetherness? Such transformative leaders are approachable, affable and available. A good leader does not boss but leads by example. Robert Greenleaf wrote the following words 50 years ago: [267]

"The servant-leader is servant first... It begins with the natural feeling that one wants to serve, to serve first. Then conscious choice brings one to aspire to lead. That person is sharply different from one who is leader first; perhaps because of the need to assuage an unusual power drive or to acquire material possessions...The leader-first and the servant-first are two extreme types. Between them there are shadings and blends that are part of the infinite variety of human nature."

SICK AND SCARED

"The difference manifests itself in the care taken by the servant-first to make sure that other people's highest priority needs are being served. The best test, and difficult to administer, is this: Do those served grow as persons? Do they, while being served, become healthier, wiser, freer, more autonomous, more likely themselves to become servants? And, what is the effect on the least privileged in society? Will they benefit or at least not be further deprived? "

A servant-leader looks after the welfare of employees and the community being served. He/she shares power and ensures the workers rise to their highest potential. Great health care leaders get "the pulse of the place" exactly right. She bridges the chasm between the generals (administrators) and the troops (health care workers).

Dr. Toby Cosgrove, the previous CEO at the Cleveland Clinic, introduced the concept of service and empathy in his organization. He asked all employees to think of each other and to imagine what difficulties others might be facing. He also insisted that all administrators do some clinical work, so they would not get isolated from the realities of practice and the obstacles workers faced. He also envisioned and implemented same day walk-in appointments for patients. The great leader is visible, and aware of the local scene.

Such leaders are admired. In my view, physician-administrators are better equipped to understand the world of physicians than non-clinicians because they have been there and done that.

Healthcare organizations have a deep desire to serve. They express that desire with elegant mission statements. The system which employs me, ChristianaCare, has one too.

"We serve our neighbors as respectful, expert, caring partners in their health. We do this by creating innovative, effective, affordable systems of care that our neighbors value."

These simple words have depth and warmth. It is not accidental that the word "neighbor" is used instead of the "patient". It creates a sense of community and feels less transactional. But how do leaders put these words into action?

One CEO I knew went to a physicians' practice to apologize personally for the bullying and inflammatory actions of one of his senior administrators. The offending official was removed from office shortly thereafter. The same CEO saw the hardship of physician lives and urged the organization to transform in order to make things "easier and better" for everyone. He also scheduled a "meet the CEO session" and "walk with the CEO" session every two weeks; open to anyone who wanted to chat with him. Very few, unfortunately, took up his offer.

Another CEO heard that her workers were sometimes doing two jobs to put food on the table for their families. She authorized a free food pantry. Any employee could use their badge, enter and take what they needed without questions, signatures, or humiliation. She also raised the minimum wage for all employees to $15 an hour, the first in the state to do so. She invested in downtrodden areas of the city to address some of the social determinants of health and increased diversity in hiring. She also allowed employees to take a paid day off for community service, encouraged a blameless but accountable system of Just Culture to pervade through the system and created a center for wellbeing. She instituted an alumni fund for residents in need (yes, there are young doctors in deep debt and facing significant hardships); saved the careers of several residents from Hahnemann University in Philadelphia when it suddenly shut down; and she funded the activities of a group seeking to address the needs of late career physicians. The program was set up to help transitioning late career physicians, nurse practitioners and physician assistants plan their futures.

And she took a knee to protest the killing of George Floyd by rogue policemen.

At the same institution, "No Pass Zones" were created where patients could expect help from any employee passing by, whether assigned to the patient or not. "Quiet at night" goals were instituted to include lights being turned down at night and TVs turned off so patients could rest. Nurses made hourly rounds to check on patients. And for those who were dying without any family or friends and who craved for company, volunteers sat by their bedside in a program called

SICK AND SCARED

"No one dies alone". Patient advisors were appointed to panels. A program (CANDOR) to disclose harm to patient and families truthfully was unveiled, becoming one of the few in the nation to do so.

During the COVID-19 crisis, health care workers were put up in pre-paid hotel rooms if they did not wish to go home and risk transmitting infection to their family members. And since all childcare centers were closed, the CEO contracted with several private centers to look after the children of health care workers at the hospital (all costs covered). There were no furloughs, and no salary reductions. A respectful dialogue was initiated to decide how to manage the fiscal gap created by the pandemic. Great institutions take care of their patients and their employees.

When the day ends, each person must ask themselves:

"What did I learn today?

How did I make a difference in the lives of the sick and scared?

Have I achieved the goals of healing those who suffer?"

If the answer is yes, be proud and keep plodding on. We have much work to do. We can and must do it and fulfill our dreams as we take care of the most vulnerable in society.

I repeat Hubert Humphrey's unforgettable words:

"Compassion is not weakness, and concern for the unfortunate is not socialism."

APPENDIX A

How we got the health care system we have: A brief history of Government programs in the US.

An act resembling Social Security (SS) was first passed in 1776, even before the declaration of independence, to help disabled soldiers and families. Civil war pensions and benefits to veterans and their survivors were granted between 1870 and 1910. The Veterans Administration came into being in 1930. It ensured that those who bear the wounds of battle are cared for. Social Security, as we know it today, became law in 1935 and millions now depend on it for survival.

President Harry Truman proposed wider access to health care, but the American Medical Association (AMA)-concerned about physician incomes-vehemently opposed the idea.

Lyndon Johnson declared a War on Poverty on January 8, 1964 and signed the Medicare bill into law in 1965 which, along with Social Security benefits, have become vital programs for the elderly, retired or disabled.

Ronald Reagan, fearing waste and rationing, rejected the idea of "socialized medicine" as an intrusion of government into private matters during the Cold War era.

Bill Clinton's health care goals fell apart due to partisan politics and resentment that Hillary Clinton, then the first lady, was chosen to lead instead of a health care expert.

The Affordable Care Act (ACA) became the law of the nation on March 23, 2010. The bill passed after several compromises and a willingness to accept something less than perfect. Twenty million of the 50 million uninsured were now covered. Americans, by wide margins, support the ACA provisions to allow students to stay on a parent's insurance until age 26; to forbid denials for pre- existing conditions and to expand coverage for the poor through Medicaid. However, the ACA did not -and could not- address the massive profits of corporations because of their stranglehold on the political process. In fact, the insurance industry agreed to the plan only because of a massive subsidy of billions of dollars granted to them to support the proposed lower premiums. Opponents derisively called the plan Obamacare. The President, with characteristic flair, pushed back by changing the phrase to "Obama Cares"!

Political opponents vowed to overturn the ACA claiming that the mandate which forces everyone to buy insurance, with penalties for noncompliance, is unconstitutional and the courts agreed. Encouraged, opponents want to scrap the entire bill. It is hard to understand the court decision because car insurance works that way too. Everyone must have car insurance whether you have ever had an accident or not. Health care for the vulnerable and unfortunate would not be possible if the majority- typically younger working citizens- did not subsidize such care through higher taxes or premiums for mandatory health care policies. The ACA's fate, as of this date, remains uncertain.

Americans are basically good and decent people but do not like being told what to do by government. Their charity comes from the heart, and they resent it when forced into a cause they may not support. Their anxiety must be acknowledged and respected. However, this rugged individualism sometimes collides with our societal obligations towards the weak, sick and dispossessed. All the data suggests that health care will be less expensive and higher in quality than what we have now if we embrace universal health care with single pay.

Critics of current government programs- Social Security, Medicare and the Veterans Administration (VA) - should ask themselves the following questions: Have these programs been in our national interest? Have they served us well? If not, should we abolish all three? Are we able or willing to give up those benefits? Are they examples of "socialism"?

As a recipient of Medicare and Social Security benefits, I have never missed a check, bill or statement from either agency over the past 12 years. Social security deducts my Medicare premiums. The free annual Medicare wellness check reminds me of cancer screening, vaccinations, blood pressure checks, screenings for depression, audiovisual problems etc.

Federal pensioners receive their checks by direct deposit as scheduled without error. The US Postal Service, a heavily subsidized mail service, handles billions of packages daily and contrary to what I read, I have rarely lost an item in 50 years.

VA hospitals, owned, operated and financed by the Government in a single payer system fare better in almost every measurement of health care outcomes and cost compared to the private system, a free market, and multi-payer, "capitalistic" enterprise. The VA is brutally criticized for its lapses and long lines -for good reason- but private institutions typically escape public scrutiny about access. VA employees are silenced. The private sector utilizes sleek external affairs departments, posts huge billboards on highways and manages the fallout from embarrassing issues. I know of waiting periods of several months simply to get an initial appointment at several major private hospitals. (Full disclosure: I spent 25 years in the VA system and almost 10 years in a private group practice/ hospital setting).

Many Americans, including doctors in the private sector, believe that VA care- a form of "socialism"- is inferior to the private sector and that VA employees are people who could not get better jobs. The data suggests otherwise. This perception is bolstered by sensational stories by TV anchors. All evidence supports the conclusion that the VA provides quality care at lower cost for a vulnerable population of veterans who have served our country well. A great majority of veterans are happy with the care they get. The VA has come closer to achieving the Triple Aim than the private sector has. I have been unable to find any research which shows the opposite.

A Stanford study showed that for matched populations of patients with kidney diseases at a similar stage, 82% of patients in the private sector got dialysis vs 53% in the VA group. This suggests that non-veterans might be getting dialysis prematurely without trying other treatment strategies first. At first glance, it might appear that people getting dialysis earlier is a good thing. However, hemodialysis for most patients requires a trip to a medical center for 3-4 hours three times a week and the quality of their life is quite miserable. Depression is common. They are usually unable to work. Their schedules revolve around the machines and there is little evidence that earlier dialysis prolongs life. Additionally, the authors reported that patients in the private sector got dialysis despite advanced dementia or metastatic disease more frequently.[268]

Dr. Ashish Jha, now the Dean at Brown University, co-authored a study with Kenneth Kizer, the Secretary of the VA in the mid-1990s and the architect of a major reengineering program within that system. It concluded that care in the VA system during 1997-2000 improved substantially from the period 1994-95 and was significantly better than that in the Medicare fee-for-service program in the private sector for 17 important indicators. [269]

O'Hanlon et al reviewed 69 studies and concluded that "The VA often (but not always) performs better than or similarly to other systems of care with regard to the safety and effectiveness of care...."[270]

Trivedi et al reviewed 36 studies to compare quality data for VA and non-VA hospitals. The conclusion: VA adherence to accepted guidelines was greater; care processes after acute myocardial infarction and processes for diabetes management were better. Mortality was similar.[271] Anhang et al reached similar conclusions.[272]

In 2003, I left a small university-affiliated VA hospital and joined a private subspecialty group associated with a 1,000-bed university affiliated private nonprofit hospital. The huge differences in the two systems were shocking. I chronicled that experience in my 2017 memoir "The Place of Cold Water."[273]

The VA system was decades ahead of the private sector with electronic records but without the administrative, chart documentation or billing distractions. At my VA facility, the clinical staff could focus on patient care. Most services were provided within one building. The private hospital in contrast used paper records, had poor care coordination and significant safety issues. The private practice model was a pressure cooker where volume, competition, productivity, profitability, billing, coding and speed were essential ingredients. Private physicians, unlike those in the VA, were hurried and harried. Bonuses depended on whether the partner was as "productive" as others in the practice. The VA has no such financial incentives.

Health care should not become a political football. Labels or buzzwords such as socialism do not serve our people well. Whatever we call a new system, it needs to be simpler, kinder, and more honest.

APPENDIX B

The Importance of International Medical graduates (IMG)

"Brown immigration" to the US began after the passage of the Civil Rights Act. For decades, the medical establishment, consisting mostly of white men, discriminated against foreign medical graduates (FMG), now labeled International Medical graduates (IMG) and especially those who came from nonwhite nations. Only some of the anxiety about language barriers -accent, command of the language and the quality of their training- was understandable. Americans are generally unaware of the high caliber of many IMG and Doctors of Osteopathy (D.O.). Both groups have faced discrimination. So even if the recruiting physicians preferred Americans, the expansion of training programs mandated that foreign medical graduates and D.O. be accepted by "weaker" training programs.

During the Vietnam era, the IMGs, legal immigrants, were eligible to be drafted and paid taxes but were denied internships in most university programs in an orchestrated manner. The rejections were predetermined, but some programs sent interview invitations to these applicants anyway to avoid any potential legal hassles. Invited doctors with limited resources would borrow money for traveling and for buying a cheap suit only to receive a predetermined rejection letter.

The foreign discards somehow got into mediocre training programs where they did much of the tedious grunt work, passed the appropriate board examinations and often became distinguished professors at the very institutions that had rejected them. They then taught the next generation of American medical students!

IMGs represent 30% of all US physicians. Clinical outcomes for graduates of US schools and IMGs are similar.[274] IMGs now outperform US trained doctors (MD or DO) in Step 1 of the United States Medical Licensing Exam (USMLE). There is a national "matching system" to allow hospitals and potential candidates to find compatible matches. Despite their higher scores, chances of an IMG matching in a coveted specialty Like ENT or orthopedics or a "high profile" training program are much lower. That is why there are disproportionately higher number of IMGs in less competitive primary care specialties (family medicine and internal medicine). This structural hierarchy is addressed in depth by the sociologist Tania Jenkins in her book *Doctor's Orders: The Making of Status Hierarchies in an Elite Program*.[275]

International Medical graduates from India have excellent clinical skills and rigorous training. Admission to Indian medical and engineering schools is extremely competitive.

Full disclosure — I am an Asian IMG, trained in a century-old medical school in India. Asian IMG now represents 18% of all doctors in the US. Abraham Verghese and I, both IMGs, have described the discrimination we experienced in the books we authored earlier.[273, 276, 277] Patients will have a hard time finding a doctor if they use race, religion, skin color or national origin as criteria for selection. In an era of significant cross coverage, one may *have* to see an "undesirable" colored, black, brown, Muslim, Hindu, Jewish, Sikh -or horror- someone with a turban or a hijab. Predominantly cognitive specialties including my own (Infectious Diseases) and Nephrology, which are more like primary care practices, are unable to fill all their training spots because of market forces. They are vital to health care but do not pay as much as surgical specialties. At least some of those training slots are being rescued by IMGs.

Many IMGs come on temporary H1-B visas, pay taxes and hope that permanent residency and citizenship will follow. This vital pipeline is shrinking because of the proposed- or feared- changes in immigration laws and long delays in processing applications. They are going to Australia, Germany, UK and New Zealand instead. US born students

SICK AND SCARED

of Asian origin are entering American medical schools in record numbers. They speak and act like "regular Americans." A patient would not be well served if he/she chose a PCP based on race, religion or national origin

APPENDIX C

CROOKS WITHIN HEALTH CARE

Diversicare Health Services, a nursing home chain in Tennessee, was fined $9.5 million for inflating bills inappropriately for Medicare Rehabilitation Services.[278]

A doctor in San Diego, Egisto Salerno, wrote prescriptions for oxycodone to homeless, incarcerated, non-existent and even dead patients "brought in by hired recruiters." They received the pills for cash. Rajendra Bhayani, an ENT surgeon, was fined $1.1 million for engaging in kickbacks with medical management companies. It was alleged that he was doing unnecessary allergy tests.[279]

Dr. Chang-Wen Chen paid $285,000 to settle allegations that he billed Medicare and Tennessee Care at the higher physician rates when the work was really done by a NP.[280]

Reinaldo and Jean Wilson who own Advantage Choice Care and Tele Medicare defrauded Medicare to the tune of $56 million by allegedly receiving illegal kickbacks and bribes from pharmacies, medical brace suppliers and patient recruiters to order medically unnecessary braces for Medicare beneficiaries from March 2017 to April 2019.[281]

On Feb 24, 2020, Dr. Mark Tamarin, a urologist from California was sentenced to 71 months in prison for fraudulently billing Medicare to the tune of $700,000. Not only did he order unnecessary tests too often before seeing patients, but he also billed for services from two locations at the same time![282]

Dr. Jorge Zamora-Quezada, a rheumatologist in Texas, falsely diagnosed patients as having rheumatoid arthritis and treated them with toxic drugs including chemotherapy. His victims included the young, old and disabled. The fraud cost Medicare $325 million. He was convicted and awaits sentencing.[283]

Ted Cain and his wife Julie Cain, defrauded Medicare of $10.8 million through fraudulent cost reports from 2004-2015. Mr. Cain requested $17.7 million in compensation even though he did no Medicare work and his wife fraudulently received more than $850,000 for administrative and consulting fees.[284]

Dr. Michael Ligotti was charged with conspiracy to commit health care fraud. He billed for fraudulent tests and services through a private clinic he owned. He served as the medical director for 50 addiction facilities and wrote 135 standing orders. In exchange for these signatures, the facilities were required to refer the patients to Ligotti. Some patients were charged $10,000 to $20,000 for a single visit. Through the alleged scheme, which ran from May 2011 through March 2020, private insurance companies and Medicare were fraudulently billed approximately $681 million. The insurers paid about $121 million of those claims, according to the Justice Department.[285]

Dr. Moses D. de Graft-Johnson is charged with stealing $26 million from Medicare, Medicaid and others for services not provided. He claimed to have done 14 procedures in 7 hours, which would normally take 28 hours. And he also billed for 13 operations in the US when he was out of the country. The stated reason for the fraud was to fund his campaign to become the President of Ghana![286]

Dr. Paul Mathieu was hired by a non-physician to pose as the owner of three clinics and falsely claimed he examined and treated patients; falsified and created phony records; and wrote prescriptions for unneeded items such as diapers and incontinence products which were then supplied by the real owner of these phony clinics.[287]

SICK AND SCARED

The University of New Mexico (UNM) in Albuquerque is being sued by 243 patients because an oncologist allegedly prescribed substandard concentrations of chemotherapy to patients with Acute Lymphocytic Leukemia over a 10-year period, increasing the risk of relapse and death. This continued despite a review by outside experts who had informed the pediatric oncology program that it was not "employing standard protocols". Survival rates were 50% at UNM vs 70% nationally. The oncologist was suspended and retired in 1997, ten years after the outside expert review.[288]

Ciox Health and several Montana hospitals were sued by four patients for charging exorbitant fees to get copies of their own records. For example, Briana Frasier, was billed a $15.00 "basic" fee, $0.50 a page fee (the legally allowed amount) and a $56.80 shipping fee *even though the record was sent electronically.*[289]

Elizabeth Rosenthal, in her book," *An American Sickness*," gives a detailed account of how pharmaceutical companies, device makers and pharmacy benefit managers make deals, bribe physicians to prescribe their products in the US and abroad, how they violate the spirit of rules and laws, stifle competition; prolong patents, sway patients with slick TV commercials and lure them with coupons and rebates for overpriced drugs.[50]

Novartis just settled a lawsuit for $678M for bribing physicians. "The pharmaceutical company spent more than $100 million on lavish meals, fishing junkets, golf outings, sporting events and speaker fees to influence doctors to prescribe its drugs, federal prosecutors said."[290]

A nurse in the ER regularly stole a portion of narcotic doses meant for patients for personal use. She then injected the rest into the patient's IV tubing. The nurse, who had an unusual form of hepatitis C, transmitted the infection to numerous patients. Elet Neilson lost her license and was sentenced to five years in prison.[291]

BIBLIOGRAPHY

1.   Montori, Victor. *Why we revolt: A patient revolution for careful and kind care*. Rochester: The Patient revolution, 2017.

2.   Case, Angela and Angus Deaton. "The Sickness of Our System: Health Care Costs Undermine Working Class Lives." *Time Magazine,* March 2-9, 2020, p 80-81

3.   Case, Angela and Angus Deaton, *Deaths of Despair and the Future of Capitalism.* Princeton: University Press, 2020

4.   Reinhart R.J. "Nurses Continue to Rate Highest in Honesty, Ethics." *Gallup Poll,* January 6, 2020.
   https://news.gallup.com/poll/274673/nurses-continue-rate-highest- honesty-ethics.aspx?versi...

5.   Wible, Pamela. *Human Rights Violations in Medicine: A-to-Z Action Guide*. Eugene, Oregon: Pamela Wible MD Publishing, 2019

6.   Sutcliffe, Kathleen. "The Health Care Industry Needs to Be More Honest About Medical Errors." *Time Magazine,* Nov 05, 2019.
   https://time.com/5717545/medical-errors/

7. Sutcliffe, Kathleen and Robert Wears. *Still Not Safe: Patient Safety and the Middle-Managing of American Medicine*. New York: Oxford University Press, 2020.

8. Source of data: Bureau of Labor Statistics; NCHS; and Himmelstein/Woolhandler analysis of CPS.

9. Dhand, Suneel. "Physicians have been given weed killer. Administrators have been given Miracle- Gro." *KevinMD*, December 22, 2019. https://kevinmd.com/blog/2019/12/physicians-have-been-given-weed-killer-admini...

10. Miller, Lee J. and Wei Lu. "These Are the World's Healthiest Nations." *Bloomberg Healthiest Country Index 2019*. February 24, 2019. https://www.bloomberg.com/news/articles/2019-02-24/spain-tops-italy-as-world-s-healthiest-nation-while-u-s-slips...

11. Newman, Katelyn. "Spain Is Considered Healthiest Country, According to New Report. The United States didn't come close to the top of the Bloomberg Healthiest Country Index." *US World and News Report*, Feb 26th, 2019.

12. Tikkanen, Roosa and Melinda K. Abrams. "U.S. Health Care from a Global Perspective, 2019: Higher Spending, Worse Outcomes?" *The Commonwealth Fund*, January 30, 2020 https://www.commonwealthfund.org/publications/issue-briefs/2020/jan/us-health-care-global-perspective-2019

13. Makary, Martin. *The Price We Pay: What Broke American Health Care- And How to Fix It*. New York: Bloomsbury Publishing, New York, 2019.

14. Makary, Martin and Daniel Michael. "Medical Error-The Third Leading Cause of Death in the US." *BMJ* 2016; 353: i2139 https://www.bmj.com/content/353/bmj.i2139.full.print

15. Topol, Eric. "Just what the doctor ordered: How AI will change medicine in the 2020s." *The Globe and Mail*, December 27, 2019. https://www.theglobeandmail.com/opinion/article-just-what-the-doctor-ordered-how-ai-will-change-medicine-in-the-2020s/

16. Topol, Eric. "Why doctors should organize." *New Yorker*, August 5, 2019. https://www.newyorker.com/culture/annals-of-inquiry/why-doctors-should-organize

17. Frellick, Marcia. "National Residents' Union Drafts Bill of Rights." *Medscape*, February 28, 2020. https://www.medscape.com/viewarticle/925930

18. The Triple Aim. Institute for Healthcare Improvement. http://www.ihi.org/engage/initiatives/TripleAim/Pages/default.aspx

19. Bodenheimer, Thomas and Christine Sinsky. "From Triple to Quadruple aim: Care of the Patient Requires Care of the Provider." *Ann Fam Med* 12, no.6 (Nov-Dec 2014): 573-6

20. Stillman, Michael and Monalisa Tailor. "Dead man walking." *New Engl J Med* 369; (2013) 1880-1881

21. Schulte, Gabriela. "What America is thinking." *The Hill*, April 19-20, 2019. https://thehill.com/hilltv/what-americas-thinking/494602-poll-69-percent-of-voters-support-medicare-for-all

22. Pearl, Robert. *Mistreated: Why We Think We're Getting Good Health Care-And Why We're Usually Wrong.* New York: Perseus Books LLC, 2017.

23. Hecht, Eric M., Marnie R Layton, Gary A Abrams, Anna M Rabil and David C Landy. "Healthy Behavior Adherence: The National Health and Nutrition Examination Survey, 2005-2016." *Am J Prev Med* 59, no. 2 April 2020) 270-273 DOI: 10.1016/j.amepre.2020.02.013

24. Ganguli, Ishani, Zhuo Shi, Aarti Rao, Kristin N. Ray and Ateev Mehrotra. "Declining Use of Primary Care among Commercially Insured Adults in the United States, 2008-2016." *Ann Intern Med* 172, (2020) 240-247. Doi: 10.7326/M19-1834.

25. Knight, Victoria. "America to face a shortage of primary care physicians within a decade or so." *The Washington Post*, July 15, 2019. https://www.washingtonpost.com/health/america-to-face-a-shortage-of-primary-care-physicians-within-a-decade-or-so/2019/07/12/0cf144d0-a27d-11e9-bd56-eac6bb02d01d_story.html

26. Cardoza, Kavitha. "Why 36 million American adults can't read enough to work — and how to help them." *PBS report*, Jun 11, 2019. https://www.pbs.org/newshour/show/why-36-million-american-adults-cant-read-enough-to-work-and-how-to-help-them

27. Tannen, Deborah. *You Just Don't Understand: Women and Men in Conversation.* New York: Ballantine Books, 1990.

28. Parker-Pore, Tara. "Should You Choose a Female Doctor?" *The New York Times,* August 14, 2018.

https://www.nytimes.com/2018/08/14/well/doctors-male-female-women-men-heart.html

29. Baumhakel, Magnus, Ulrike Muller and Michael Bohm. "Influence of gender of physicians and patients on guideline-recommended treatment of chronic heart failure in a cross-sectional study." *Eur J Heart Fail* 11, no. 3 (Mar 2009): 299-303

30. Berthold H.K., I. Gouni-Berhtold, K.P. Bestehorn, M. Bohm and W. Krone. "Physician gender is associated with the quality of Type 2 diabetes care." *J Intern Med* 264, no. 4 (Oct 2008): 340-50 doi:10.1111/j.1365-2796.2008.01967. X.

31. Jones, Rada. "Why choose a woman doctor?" *KevinMD*. Nov 20, 2019 https://www.kevinmd.com/blog/2019/11/why-choose-a-woman-doctor.html

32. Tsugawa Y., J.P. Newhouse, A.M. Zaslavsky, D. M. Blumenthal, A. B. Jena. "Physician Age and Outcomes in elderly patients in hospital in the US: observational study." *BMJ* 2017; 357: j1797 doi: 10.1136/bmj. j1797

33. Beckman, Howard B. and Richard M. Frankel. "The Effect of Physician Behavior on the Collection of Data." *Ann Intern Med* 101, no. 5 (1984) 692-696. doi:10.7326/0003-4819-101-5-692

34. Marvel, M.K., R.M. Epstein, K. Flowers, H.B. Beckman. "Soliciting the patient's agenda; have we improved?" *JAMA* 1999;281(3):283-287 doi:10.1001/jama.281.3.283

35. Singh Ospina, Naykky, Kari A. Phillips, Kari, Rene Rodriguez-Gutierrez, Ana Castaneda-Guarderas, Michael R. Gionfriddo, Megan E. Branda, and Victor M. Montori. "Eliciting the

Patient's Agenda- Secondary Analysis of Recorded Clinical Encounters." *J GEN INTERN MED* 34, 36–40 (2019). https://doi.org/10.1007/s11606-018-4540-5)

36. Verghese, Abraham. "Culture Shock-Patient as Icon, Icon as Patient." *N Engl J Med* 359, (2008) 2748-2751. doi: 10.1056/NEJMp0807461

37. Arndt, Brian G., John W. Beasley, Michelle D. Watkinson, Jonathan L. Temte, Wen-Jan Tuan, Christine A. Sinsky and Valerie J. Gilchrist. "Tethered to the EHR: Primary Care Physician Workload Assessment Using EHR Event Log Data and Time-Motion Observations." *The Annals of Family Medicine* September 2017, 15 (5) 419-426; DOI: https://doi.org/10.1370/afm.2121

38. Olson, Douglas P., and Donna M. Windish. "Communication Discrepancies between Physicians and Hospitalized Patients." *Arch Intern Med* 170, no.15 (2010) 1302-1307

39. Elena Durnbaugh. "Patient who speaks limited English turned away from appointment at Bronson Hospital." *Battle Creek Enquirer,* December 9, 2019. https://www.battlecreekenquirer.com/story/news/local/2019/12/09/patient-who-speaks-limited-english-turned-away-bronson-hospital/4353570002/

40. Lee, Thomas H. *An Epidemic of Empathy in Healthcare: How to deliver compassionate, connected patient care that creates a competitive advantage.* New York: McGraw Hill Education, 2016.

41. Koster, John, Gary Bisbee, and Ram Charan. *n=1: How the uniqueness of each individual is transforming healthcare.* Westport, CT: The Academy Press and Prospecta Press, 2014.

42. "Nebraska doctor lets patients pay for surgery by volunteering: "We want to be able to offer hope" *CBS News*, January 23, 2020. https://www.cbsnews.com/news/medical-bills-nebraska-doctor-lets-patients-pay-for-surgery-with-volunteer-service/

43. DePaulo, Bella. "Singlism: What It Is and Is Not, and Why It Should Be in the dictionary." *Psychology Today*, September 20, 2010. https://www.psychologytoday.com/us/blog/living-single/201009/singlism-what-it-is-and-is-not-and-why-it-should-be-in-the-dictionary

44. Joan DelFattore. "Death by Stereotype? Cancer treatment in Unmarried Patients." *N Engl J Med* 381, no. 10(Sept 2019): 982-5

45. Rappleye, Emily. *Becker's Hospital Review*, December 5, 2019 https://www.beckershospitalreview.com/legal-regulatory-issues/neurologist-sues-patient-fa...

46. Hospital Quality www.medicare.gov/hospitalcompare

47. Bai, Ge, Farah Yehia and Gerard F. Anderson. "Charity Care Provision by US Nonprofit Hospitals." *JAMA Intern Med* 180, no. 4. (2020): 606-607   doi:10.1001/jamainternmed.2019.7415

48. Crouch, Michelle. (Quoting Pat Palmer, CEO of Medical Billing Advocates of America). "50 secrets hospitals won't tell you." *Readers Digest*, February 2016, page 64

49. Paavola, Alia. "The 70 CMS-mandated services hospitals must post online." *Becker's Hospital Review*, February 13, 2020. https://www.beckershospitalreview.com/finance/the-70-cms-mandated-services-hospitals-...

50. Rosenthal, Elizabeth. "Analysis: In Medical Billing, Fraudulent Charges Weirdly Pass as Legal." *Kaiser Health News,* December 16, 2019. https://khn.org/news/analysis-in-medical-billing-fraudulent-charges-weirdly-pass-...

51. Source: The State Health Access Data Assistance Center, University of Minnesota as quoted by *AARP magazine,* page 40, December 2019

52. The History of a Wonderful Thing we call Insulin. The American Diabetes Association, July 1, 2019. https://www.diabetes.org/blog/history-wonderful-thing-we-call-insulin

53. Marston, Laura. "Health Policy Poets Light Up Twitter for Valentine's Day." *Medscape* - Feb 18, 2020 https://www.medscape.com/viewarticle/925372

54. Ahamed, Akram, Kimberly C. Kullmann, Rosemary Frasso and Jennifer Goldstein. "Analysis of Unregulated Sale of Life-Saving Prescription Drugs Online in the United States." *JAMA Intern Med* 180, no. 4 (February 2020): 606-609 doi:10.1001/jamainternmed.2019.7514

55. Kang, Cecilia. "Martin Shkreli Faces New Accusations Over High-Priced Drug." *New York Times,* January 27, 2020. https://www.nytimes.com/2020/01/27/business/martin-shkreli-ftc-lawsuit.html

56. Lazarus, David. "Column: Always look on the bright side of life, says CEO who raised EpiPen price by more than 400%." *Orlando*

Sentinel, June 5, 2018. http://www.orlandosentinel.com/business/la-fi-lazarus-mylan-epipen-drug-prices-20180605-story.html

57. Anderson, Maia. "Roche Pulled a $1.5B fast one on US, whistleblower physician alleges." *Becker's Hospital Review,* January 14, 2020. https://www.beckershospitalreview.com/pharmacy/roche-pulled-a-1-5b-fast-one-on-u-s-w...

58. Feldman, William B., Benjamin N. Rome, Lisa S. Lehmann and Aaron S. Kesselheim. "Estimation of Medicare Part D Spending on Insulin for Patients with Diabetes Using Negotiated Prices and a Defined Formulary." *JAMA Intern Med* 180, no. 4 (Feb 2019): 597-601 doi:10.1001/jamainternmed.2019.7018

59. Ledley, Fred D., Sarah S. McCoy, Gregory, Vaughan and Ekaterina G. Cleary. "Profitability of Large Pharmaceutical Companies Compared with Other Large Public Companies." *JAMA Intern Med* 323, no. 9 (Mar 2020): 834-843 doi:10.1001/jama.2020.0442

60. Wouters, Olivier J. "Lobbying expenditures and campaign contributions by the pharmaceutical and Health Product Industry in the United States, 1999-2018." *JAMA Intern Med* 180, no.5 (Mar 2020): 688-697 doi:10.1001/jamainternmed.2020.0146.

61. Cattanach, Jamie. "1 in 3 Cardholders Are in Credit Card Debt Due to Medical Bills." *Compare Cards,* Nov 5, 2019. https://www.comparecards.com/blog/one-third-cardholders-credit-card-debt-reason-medical-bills/

62. McArdle, Megan. "The Truth about Medical Bankruptcies." *The Washington Post,* March 26, 2018.

https://www.washingtonpost.com/blogs/post-partisan/wp/2018/03/26/the-truth-about-medical-bankruptcies...

63.   Himmelstein, David U., Terry Campbell and Steffie Woolhander. "Health Care Administrative Costs in the United States and Canada, 2017." *Ann Intern Med* 172, no. 2 (Jan 2020) 134-142 doi: 10.7326/M19-2818.

64.   Shrank, William H., Teresa L. Rogstad and Natasha Parekh. "Waste in the US Health Care System: Estimated Costs and Potential for Saving." *JAMA Intern Med* 322, no.15, (Oct 2019): 1501-1509 doi:10.1001/jama.2019.13978

65.   Berwick, Donald M. (editorial) "Elusive Waste: The Fermi Paradox in US Health Care." *JAMA Intern Med* 322, no.15 (Oct 2019): 1458-1459 doi: 10.1001/jama2019.14610

66.   Spector, Mike. "Exclusive: U.S. Pursues Nearly $13 Billion of Claims in Purdue Pharma Opioid Probes, Sources Say." *US World and News Report*, August 4, 2020. https://www.usnews.com/news/top-news/articles/2020-08-04/exclusive-us-pursues-nearly-13-billion-of-claims-in-purdue-pharma-opioid-probes-sources-say

67.   Allen, Marshall. "How One Employer Stuck a New Mom With an $898,984 Bill for Her Premature Baby." *ProPublica*, November 4, 2019 www.propublica.org/article/how-one-employer-stuck-a-new-mom-with-a-bill-for-h...

68.   Harris, Richard. "For Her Head Cold, Insurer Coughed Up $25,865." *Morning Edition, NPR* December 23, 2019. https://www.npr.org/sections/health-shots/2019/12/23/787403509/for-her-head-cold-insurer-coughed-up-25-865

69. Carreyrou, John. *Bad Blood: Secrets and Lies in a Silicon Valley Startup*. New York, Knopf, May 21, 2018. 352 pages

70. Goldstein, Jennifer, Zhang Zugui, J. Sanford Schwartz and LeRoi S. Hicks. "Observation Status, Poverty and High Financial Liability among Medicare Beneficiaries." *Am J Med* 131 no.1 (Jan 2018) 101 https://doi.org/10.1006/j.amjmed.2017.07.013

71. Taylor, Andrew. "Opinion: I'm on Medicare, but I still got stuck with a $25,000 hospital bill." *Los Angeles Times*, December 20, 2019 https://www.latimes.com/opinion/story/2019-12-20/medicare-coverage-hospitalization-patient-costs

72. "Surprising Out-of-Pocket Costs for Caregivers." *AARP Bulletin/Real Possibilities* October 2019 https://www.aarp.org/caregiving/financial-legal/info-2019/out-of-pocket-costs.html

73. Lin, Sunny C., Courtney R. Lyles, Urmimala Sarkar and Julia Adler-Milstein. "Are Patients Electronically Accessing Their Medical Records? Evidence from the National Hospital data." *Health Affairs* 38, no.11 (Nov 2019) 1850-1857

74. Wheat, Santina. "I struggle with my pride in the profession and fear of the health care system." *KevinMD*, February 29, 2020. https://www.kevinmd.com/blog/2020/02/i-struggle-with-my-pride-in-the-profession-and-fea...

75. Doty, Michelle M., Roosa Tikkanen, Arnav Shah and Eric C. Schneider. "International Survey: Primary Care Physicians in the U.S. struggle more to coordinate care and communicate with other providers but offer patients more health IT tools. 2019

Commonwealth Fund International Health Policy Survey of Primary Care Physicians." *The Commonwealth Fund.* https://www.commonwealthfund.org/publications/journal-article/2019/dec/international-s...

76. "*To Err is Human: Building a Safer Health System.*" Washington, DC: National Academy Press, Institute of Medicine, 2000. http://www.nap.edu/books/0309068371/html/ www.iom.edu

77. Studdert, David M., Michelle M. Mello, Atul A. Gawande, Troyen A. Brennan, and Y. Claire Wang. "Disclosure of Medical Injury to Patients: An Improbable Risk Management Strategy." *Health Affairs* 26, no.1 (Jan-Feb 2007): 215–226 https://www.healthaffairs.org/doi/full/10.1377/hlthaff.26.1.215https://doi.org/ 10.1377/hlthaff.26.1.215

78. Kraman, Steve S. and Ginny Hamm. "Risk management: Extreme honesty may be the best policy." *Ann Intern Med* 131, no. 12(Dec 1999): 963-967 https://doi.org/10.7326/0003-4819-131-12-199912210-00010

79. Kachalia, Allen, Samuel R. Kaufman, Richard Boothman and Susan Anderson. "Liability Claims and Costs Before and After Implementation of a Medical Error Disclosure Program." *Ann Intern Med 153*, no. 4 (Aug 2010) 213-221 https://annals.org/aim/article-abstract/745972/liability-claims-costs-before-after-implement...

80. McDonald, Timothy B., L.A. Helmchen, K.M. Smith, N. Centomani, A. Gunderson, D. Mayer and W.H. Chamberlin. "Responding to patient safety incidents: the seven pillars." *Qual Saf Health Care* 19, no.6 (2009)   doi:10.1136/qshc.2008.031633

81. "The Future of Healthcare: A National Survey of Physicians-2018." *Doctors Company report.* https://www.thedoctors.com/about-the-doctors-company/newsroom/the-future-of-healthcare-survey/

82. Gawande, Atul. "Why Doctors Hate Their Computers." *New Yorker,* November 12, 2018. https://www.newyorker.com/magazine/2018/11/12/why-doctors-hate-their-computers.

83. Srivastava, Ranjana. "When the EMR Stole My Pen." *N Engl J Med* 383, (Aug 2020):708-709 DOI: 10.1056/NEJMp2000272

84. Califf, Robert M. and R. A. Rosati. "The doctor and the computer." *West J Med* 135, no.4 (Oct 1981) 321-323

85. Verghese, Abraham, Nigam H. Shah, and Robert A. Harrington: "What this Computer Needs is a Physician. Humanism and Artificial Intelligence." *JAMA Intern Med* 319, no. 1(Dec 2017): 19-20. doi:10.1001/jama.2017.19198

86. Verghese, Abraham, Blake Charlton, Jerome Kassirer, Megan Ramsey and John P.A. Ioannidis. "Inadequacies of Physical Examination as a cause of Medical Errors and Adverse Events: A Collection of Vignettes." *Amer J Med* 128, no. 12 (Dec 2015): 1322-1324.e3 https://doi.org/10.1016/j.amjmed.2015.06.004

87. Sinsky, Christine, Lacey Colligan, Ling Li, Mirela Prgomet, Sam Reynolds, Lindsey Goeders, Johanna Westbrook, Michael Tutty and George Blike. "Allocation of Physician Time in Ambulatory Practice: A Time and Motion Study in 4 Specialties." *Ann Intern Med* 165, no. 11, (Dec 2016):753-760. doi: 10.7326/M16-0961

88. Overhage, J. Marc and David McCallie. "Physician Time Spent Using the Electronic Health Record During Patient Encounters." *Ann Intern Med* 172, no. 3 (Feb 2020) 169-174 doi:10.7326/M18-3684

89. Skolnik, Neil and Chris Notte. "Whispered pectoriloquy." *MDedge*, August 4, 2015. https://www.mdedge.com/chestphysician/article/101672/practice-management/whispered-...

90. Kostman, Jay. "Listen to your Heart- A Physician's Journey in Self-Diagnosis." *American College of Physicians*, Annual meeting, Delaware Chapter, Feb 8, 2020

91. Ellison, Ayla. "These 10 physician specialties generate the most revenue for hospitals." *Becker's Hospital Review*, May 21, 2020. www.beckershospitalreview.com/finance/these-10-physician-specialties-generate-the-most-revenue-for-hospitals

92. Popa, Rachel. "The 2018-9 physician compensation report." *Doximity*, April 2, 2019. https://blog.doximity.com/articles/doximity-2019-physician-compensation-report-d0ca91d1-3cf1-4cbb-b403-a49b9ffa849f

93. Zimmerman, Andre, Christopher Worsham, Jaemin Woo and Anupam B. Jena. "The Need for Speed: Observational study of physician driving behaviors." *BMJ* 367, l6354 (Dec 2019) https://doi.org/10.1136/bmj.l6354

94. Mulder, James T. "Free Syracuse medical clinic that served thousands of uninsured patients closes." *Syracuse.com*, November 19, 2019. https://www.syracuse.com/health/2019/11/free-syracuse-medical-clinic-that-served-thousands-of-uninsured-patients-closes.html

95. Basu, Sanjay, Russell S. Phillips, Robert Phillips, Lars E. Petersen and Bruce E. Landon. "Primary Care Finances in the United States amid the COVID-19 Pandemic." *Health Affairs* Published Online June 25, 2020 ahead of print. https://doi.org/10.1377/HLTHAFF.2020.00794

96. Shanafelt, Tait, Joel Goh and Christine Sinsky. "The Cost of Recruiting and Replacing a Physician; the Business Case for Investing in Physician Well-being." *JAMA Intern Med* 177, no. 12 (Dec 2017) 1826-1832

97. Gold, Russell and Michelle Hackman. "COVID-19 Spreads Deportation fears among Immigrant Doctors in U.S. Death and job loss from pandemic threaten visa status of physicians and families." *The Wall Street Journal*, June 1, 2020. https://www.wsj.com/articles/covid-19-spreads-deportation-fears-among-immigrant-doctors-in-u-s-11590836401

98. "Coronavirus Death of Doctor, Li Weinlang, Sparks Anger." *BBC News* February 7, 2020. https://www.bbc.com/news/world-asia-china-51409801

99. Frellick, Marcia. "Colleagues mourn Italian "Hero" Physician killed by COVID-19." *Medscape*, March 13, 2020. https://www.medscape.com/viewarticle/926816

100. Rosenthal, Elizabeth. *An American Sickness: How Healthcare Became a Business and How You can take it Back*. New York: Penguin Press, 2018.

101. Ofri, Danielle. "The business of health care depends on exploiting doctors and nurses." *New York Times*, June 8, 2019.

102. Copelan, Russel." What we get wrong about Physician Suicide-Are the stories we hear cautionary or hyperbolic?" *MedPageToday* March 9, 2020.
https://www.medpagetoday.com/blogs/suicide-watch/85310?xid=nl_blog2020-03-09&...

103. Haney, Craig, Curtis W. Banks and Philip G. Zimbardo. "A study of prisoners and guards in a simulated prison." *Naval Research Review* 30, (1973) 4-17.

104. Pies, Ronald. "Residents from Hell: Indignities and Outcomes in Medical training." *Medscape,* December 12, 2019.
https://www.medscape.com/viewarticle/922346

105. Thomas, Koren. "The Risks of Not Being Rested— How nurses can make sure they get enough sleep." *MedPagetoday,* December 29, 2019
https://www.medpagetoday.com/nursing/nursing/84121?utm_source=Sailthrou&utm_mediu...

106. Jagsi, Reshma, Kent A. Griffith, Rochelle Jones, Chithra R. Perumalswami, Peter Ubel and Abigail Stewart. "Sexual Harassment and Discrimination Experiences of Academic Medical Faculty." *JAMA* 315, no. 19 (May 2016): 2120-2121 doi:10.1001/jama.2016.2188

107. Gawande, Atul. "Big Med. Restaurant chains have managed to combine quality control, cost control, and innovation. Can health care?" *New Yorker*, August 6, 2012.
https://www.newyorker.com/magazine/2012/08/13/big-med

108. Beaulieu, Nancy D., Leemore S. Dafny, Bruce E. Landon, Jesse Dalton, Ifedayo Kuye and J. Michael McWilliams. "Changes in

Quality of Care after Hospital Mergers and Acquisitions." *N Engl J Med* 382, (Jan 2020): 51-59. DOI:10.1056/NEJMsa1901383

109. Neprash, Hannah T., Michael E Chernew, Andrew L Hicks and J Michael McWilliams. "Association of financial integration between physicians and hospitals with commercial health prices." *JAMA Intern Med* 175, no.12 (Dec 2015):1932-9 DOI: 10.1001/jamainternmed.2015.4610

110. Potter, Wendell. "After Pushing Lies, Former Cigna Executive Praises Canada's Health Care System." Interview with Michel Martin, *NPR*, on June 27, 2020.

111. Wolfson, Daniel, John Santa and Lorie Slass. "Engaging Physicians and Consumers in Conversations about Treatment Overuse and Waste. A Short History of the Choosing Wisely Campaign." *Academic Medicine* 89, no.7 (July 2014): 990-995. doi:10.1097/ACM.0000000000000270

112. Stokowski, Laura A., Mary McBride and Emily Berry. The 2019 Medscape Nurse Career Satisfaction Report. *Medscape*, December 4, 2019 https://www.medscape.com/slideshow/2019-nurse-career-satisfaction-6012376

113. Jalian, Ray H. and Mathew M. Avram. "Mid-Level Practitioners in Dermatology: A Need for Further Study and Oversight." *JAMA Dermatol* 150, no.11 (Nov 2014):1149–1151 doi:10.1001/jamadermatol.2014.1922

114. Hughes, Danny R., Miao Jiang and Richard Duszak Jr. "A Comparison of Diagnostic Imaging Ordering Patterns Between Advanced Practice Clinicians and Primary Care Physicians Following

Office-Based Evaluation and Management Visits." *JAMA Intern Med* 175, no.1 (Jan 2015):101-107 doi:10.1001/jamainternmed.2014.6349

115.   Mizrahi, Daniel, Laurence Parker, Adam M. Zogal and David C. Levin. "National Trends in the Utilization of Skeletal Radiography from 2003-2015." *J Am Coll Radiol* 15, no.10 (Oct 2018):1408-1414   doi: 10.1016/j.jacr.2017.10.007.

116.   Chen, Chiavi, Donna McNeese-Smith, Marie Cowan, Valda Upenieks and Abdelmommen Afifi. "Evaluation of a Nurse Practitioner led Care management Model in Reducing Inpatient drug Utilization and Cost." *Nursing Economics* 27, no. 3 (May-June 2009):160-168

117.   Jones, Marsha G., Linda V De Cherrie, Yasmin S. Meah, Cameron R. Hernandez, Eric J. Lee, David M. Skovran, Theresa A. Soriano and Katherine A. Ornstein. "Using Nurse Practitioner Co-Management to Reduce Hospitalization and Readmissions within a Home-based Primary Care Program." *Journal of Health Care Quality* 39, no. 5 (September-October 2017):249-258. doi:10.1097/JHQ.0000000000000059

118.   Rappleye, Emily. "28 states with full practice authority for NPs." Dec 23, 2019. https://www.beckershospitalreview.com/hospital-physician-relationships/28-states-with-full-practice-authority-for-nps.html

119.   Fiore, Kristina. "15 Doctors Fired from Chicago-Area Health System. 15 Doctors Fired from Chicago-Area Health System — Physicians "broadsided" by their termination." *MedPage Today*, November 26, 2019 https://www.medpagetoday.com/special-reports/exclusives/83576

120. Chierici, Colleen, Aney Abraham, Lynne Braun, Raechel Ferry-Rooney, Ingrid Forsberg, Terry Gallagher and Angela Moss, "Advanced nurse practitioners resent being called "mid-level" providers." Becker's Hospital Review, December 11, 2019.
https://www.beckershospitalreview.com/hospital-physician-relationships/letter-to-the-edit

121. Punjabi, Raj. "Where Neighbors provide health care, pay them." *Time Magazine* November 4, 2019.
https://time.com/5709344/governments-should-pay-community-health-workers/

122. Punjabi, Raj. Keynote Speech 3, Institute for Healthcare Improvement, December 11, 2019.

123. "History of the Physician Assistant Profession." *AAPA*
https://www.aapa.org/about/history

124. Gooch, Kelly. "Physician assistant median annual base salary, by state." *Becker's Hospital Review*, August 2020
https://www.beckershospitalreview.com/compensation-issues/physician-assistant-median-

125. Christensen, Clayton M., Jerome H. Grossman, and Jason Hwang. *The Innovator's Prescription: A Disruptive Solution for Health Care.* New York: McGraw-Hill, 2009.

126. Phillips, Robert L., Andrew W. Bazemore, Warren P. Newton. "Medical Professionalism: A contract with Society." *The Pharos*, Autumn 2019, pp 2-7
https://alphaomegaalpha.org/pharos/2019/Autumn/19_Autumn_Editorial.pdf

127. Lopatin, Mark. "The Devaluation of Physicians." *KevinMD* June 19, 2019. https://www.kevinmd.com/blog/2019/06/the-devaluation-of-physicians.html

128. Brightman, Baird. "3 reasons why doctors don't unionize." *KevinMD*, July 10, 2020. https://www.kevinmd.com/blog/2020/07/3-reasons-why-doctors-dont-unionize.html

129. "Fostering Productive Heath Care Cost Conversations: Sharing Lessons Learned and Best Practices." *Ann Intern Med* 170, no. 9 (May 2019): ACP supplement

130. DelFattore, Joan. "Please, doctor, don't rush on my account." *KevinMD*, January 31, 2017. https://www.kevinmd.com/blog/2017/01/please-doctor-dont-rush-account.html

131. Frellick, Marcia." The Medscape Malpractice Report." *Medscape,* November 21, 2019. www.medscape.com/viewarticle/921706

132. Bruce Y. Lee. "Will Ohio Bill Force Doctors to Do the Impossible: Re-implant Ectopic Pregnancies?" *Forbes*, December 2, 2019. https://www.forbes.com/sites/brucelee/2019/12/02/will-ohio-bill-force-doctors-to-do-the-impossible-reimplant-ectopic-pregnancies/#4ae19cd84948

133. Long, Heather. "Every American family basically pays an $8,000 'poll tax' under the U.S. health system, top economists." *The Seattle Times,* Jan 2020. https://www.seattletimes.com/nation-world/nation/every-american-family-basically-pays-an-8000-poll-tax-under-the-u-s-health-system-top-economists-say/

134. David Marx. "Patient Safety and the Just Culture." *Obstetrics and Gynecology Clinics of North America* 46, no. 2 (June 2019) 239-245

135. WHO International Classification of Diseases diagnostic manual. June 2018. https://www.who.int/classifications/en/

136. Talbot Simon G., and Wendy Dean. "Physicians aren't "burning out." They are suffering from moral injury." *Stat News*, July 2018. https://www.statnews.com/2018/07/26/physicians-not-burning-out-they-are-suffering-moral...

137. "Physician Burnout Survey." June 2019 www.incrowdnow.com

138. Samuel Shem. *The House of God*. New York: Richard Marek Publishers, August 30, 1978 (1st ed.)

139. Brazeau, Chantal M.L.R., Tait D. Shanafelt, Steven J. Durning, Massie F. Stanford, Anne Eaker, Christine Moutier, Daniel V. Satele et al "Distress among matriculating medical students relative to the general population." *Acad Med* 89, no. 11 (Nov 2014): 1520-1525 doi:10.1097/ACM.0000000000000482

140. West, Colin P., Liselotte N. Dyrbye and Tait D. Shanafelt. "Physician burnout: contributors, consequences and solutions." *J of Internal Medicine* 283, no. 6, (June 2018): 516-529, https://doi.org/10.1111/joim.12752

141. Kay, Adam. *This Is Going to Hurt: Secret Diaries of a Junior Doctor*. London: Picador, 2017.

142. Yellowlees, Peter M. "Why Is Physician Well-being Declining? It's the System, Stupid." *Medscape Psychiatry*, September 06, 2019 https://www.medscape.com/viewarticle/917693

143. Mehta, Nisha. "Physician Burnout: Why it is not about resilience-much more a "stress fracture" than an "insufficiency fracture." *MedPageToday*. April 26, 2018. https://medpagetoday.com/publichealthpolicy/generalprofessionalissues/72551

144. Sinsky, Christine A. "Designing and regulating wisely: Removing Barriers to Joy in Practice." *Ann Intern Med* 166, no.9 (May 2017): 677-8

145. Krasner, Michael S. Ronald M. Epstein, Howard Beckman, Anthony L. Suchman, Benjamin Chapman, Christopher J. Mooney and Timothy E. Quill. "Association of an Educational program in Mindful Communication with burnout, Empathy, and attitudes Among primary Care Physicians." *JAMA Intern Med* 302, no.12 (Sept 2009): 1284-1293   doi:10.1001/jama.2009.1384

146. Jha, Ashish K., Andrew R. Iliff, Alain A. Chaoui, Steven Defossez, Mryann C. Bombaugh and Yael R. Miller. "A Crisis in Health Care. A Call to Action on Physician Burnout from the MMA-MHA (Mass Medical Society and Mass Health and Hospital Association) Joint Task Force on Physician Burnout." 2018 www.massmed.org/News.../Physician-Burnout-Report-2018

147. Caplan, Arthur- "Is the Wellness Industry Friend or Faux?" *Medscape*, November 19, 2019. www.medscape.com/viewarticle/920109

148. Su, Leonard. "All the Wellness in the World won't help physician burnout." *KevinMD*, October 26, 2019. https://www.kevinmd.com/blog/2019/10/all-the...

149. Vaidya, Anuja. "11 ways physicians cope with burnout." *Becker's Hospital Review*, Jan 31, 2020 https://www.beckershospitalreview.com/hospital-physician-relationships/11-ways-physicians-cope-with-burnout.html

150. Silverman, Mark E., T. Jock Murray and Charles S. Bryan ed., *The Quotable Osler* (revised edition). The American College of Physicians, Versa Press, 2008

151. Dellinger EP, C.A. Pellegrini CA and Timothy Gallagher. "The Aging Physician and the Medical Profession. A Review." *JAMA Surgery* doi:10.1001/jamasurg.2017.2342.

152. "Statement on the Aging Surgeon" by the American College of Surgeons, Online January 1, 2016. https://www.facs.org/about-acs/statements/80-aging-surgeon

153. Cooney, Leo and Thomas Balcezak. "Cognitive Testing of Older Clinicians Prior to Recredentialing." *JAMA* 323, no. 2 (Jan 2020):179-180   doi:10.1001/jama.2019.18665

154. Press Release 02-11-2020. "EEOC Sues Yale New Haven Hospital for Age and Disability Discrimination." https://www.eeoc.gov/newsroom/eeoc-sues-yale-new...

155. Tony Hsieh. *Delivering Happiness*. New York: Grand Central Publishing, 2010.

156. Gallegos, Alex. "Doctor Wins $4.75 Million in Defamation Suit against Hospital." *Medscape*, January 28, 2020 https://www.medscape.com/viewarticle/924386

157. West, Melanie Grayce. "SUNY Downstate Accused of Retaliating Against Whistleblower Surgeons." *The Wall Street Journal*, Jan. 22, 2020 https://www.wsj.com/articles/suny-downstate-accused-of-retaliating-against.

158. Swanson, Conrad and Jessica Seaman. "Council members unhappy about Denver Health's executive bonuses — from $29,000 to more than $230,000." *The Denver Post*, April 29, 2020. https://www.denverpost.com/2020/04/29/denver-health-council-executive-bonuses-coronavirus/

159. Paavola, Alia. "3 Texas health systems settle lawsuit alleging they colluded to stifle nurse pay. *Becker's Hospital Review*, Jan 22, 2020. https://www.beckershospitalreview.com/legal-regulatory-issues/3-texas-health-systems-set...

160. Dulaney, H.G., and Edward Hake Phillips. *Speak, Mister Speaker*. Bonham, Texas: Sam Rayburn Foundation, 1978. p138. (Sam Rayburn used this phrase during a filmed conversation with reporters in 1953)

161. Rosenbaum, Lisa. "Costs, Benefits, and Sacred Values — Why Health Care Reform Is So Fraught." *N Engl J Med* 382, no. 2 (Jan 2020):101-104   doi: 10.1056/NEJMp1916615

162. Gawande, Atul. *Better: A Surgeon's notes on Performance*. New York: Henry Holt; 2008

163. "Better is Possible: The American College of Physicians' Vision for the U.S. Health Care System." *Ann Intern Med* 172, no. 2 (supplement) Jan 21, 2020

164. John Conyers' Bill 676.
https://www.congress.gov/bill/115th-congress/house-bill/676

165. Call for health care for all by the American Association of Family Practitioners.
https://www.aafpfoundation.org/content/dam/foundation/documents/who-we-are/cfhm/factsonfile/AAFPChronology.pdf

166. Haefner, Morgan. 16 medical groups that support 'Medicare for All,' single payer. *Becker's Hospital Review*, January 22, 2020.
https://www.beckershospitalreview.com/payer-issue/16-medical-groups-that-support-med...

167. Lindmark, Augie W., Micah A Johnson and Alec M Feuerbach. "Doctors and Dark Money: A Bad Prescription for Health Reform." *Medscape*, March 6, 2020
https://www.medscape.com/viewarticle/926307

168. Fuchs, Victor. "Is single Payer System the Answer for the US Health Care System?" *JAMA* 319, no. 1 (Jan 2018) :15-16. doi:10.1001/jama.2017.18739

169. Medicare Strike Force oig.hhs.gov

170. Levine, Hallie. "What to Know about Concierge Medicine; a doctor who has time to talk to you can be yours — for a price." *AARP*, April 25, 2019

171. Stillman, Michael. "Concierge Medicine: A 'Regular' Physician's Perspective." *Ann Intern Med* 152, no.6 (Mar 2010):391-392 https://doi.org/10.7326/0003-4819-152-6-201003160-00009

172. Risa, Kathleen J., Lisa Nepon, Janice C. Justis, Anand Panwalker, Stephen M. Berman, Sandro Cinti, Marilyn M. Wagener and Nina Singh. "Alternative therapy use in HIV-infected patients receiving highly active antiretroviral therapy." *Int J STD AIDS* 13, no. 10(Oct 2002):706-13

173. Ellison, Ayla. "Medicare to cover acupuncture for low back pain." *Becker's Hospital Review*, January 21, 2020. https://www.beckershospitalreview.com/finance/medicare-to-cover-acupuncture-for-chroni…

174. Garrity, Mackenzie. 10 updates on Amazon's healthcare push. *Becker's Hospital Review*, Dec 6, 2019 https://www.beckershospitalreview.com/consumerism/10-updates-on-amazon-s-healthcare…

175. Niran S. Al-Agba, "Delivering health care at a retail clinic isn't something to be proud of." August 9, 2020. *KevinMD*, https://www.kevinmd.com/blog/2020/08/delivering-health-care-at-a-retail-clinic-isnt-something-to-be-proud-of.html

176. Wachter, Robert M. and Lee Goldman. "Perspective-Zero to 50,000 — the 20th Anniversary of the Hospitalist." *N Engl J Med* 375 (2016): 1009-1011   DOI:10.1056/NEJMp1607958

177. What Is the Average Hospitalist Salary by State in 2020? https://www.ziprecruiter.com/Salaries/What-Is-the-Average-Hospitalist-Salary-by-State.

178. Goodwin, James S., Shuang Li and Yong-Fang Kuo. "Association of the Work Schedules of Hospitalists with Patient Outcomes of Hospitalization." *JAMA Intern Med* 180, no.2 (Feb 2020) 215-222 doi:10.1001/jamainternmed.2019.5193

179. Lee, Robert Y. Lyndia C. Brumback, Seelwan Sathitratanacheewin, Lober, William B., Modes, Mathew E., Lynch, Ylinne T., Ambrose et al "Association of Physician Orders for Life-Sustaining Treatment with ICU Admission Among Patients Hospitalized Near the End of Life." *JAMA Intern Med* 323, no. 10 (Feb 2020): 950-960 doi:10.1001/jama.2019.22523

180. Moore-Black, Debbie. When a wife won't let her husband die. *KevinMD*, February 27, 2020. https://www.kevinmd.com/blog/2020/02/when-a-wife-wont-let-her-husband-die.html

181. Barnett, Michael L., Andrew R. Olenski and Anupam B. Jena. "Patient Mortality during Unannounced Accreditation Surveys at US Hospitals." *JAMA Intern Med* 177, no. 5 (Mar 2017): 693-700 doi:10.1001/jamainternmed.2016.9685

182. Han, Lu, Matt Sutton, Stuart Clough, Richard Warner and Tim Doran. "Impact of Out-of-Hours Admission on patient mortality: longitudinal analysis in a tertiary acute hospital." *BMJ Qual Saf* 27, no. 6 (June 2018):445-454   doi:10.1136/bmjqs-2017-006784

183. Top ten best countries for medical tourism and overseas healthcare. http://sleepredeye.com/uncategorized/top-10-best-countries-for-medical-tourism-and-overseas-healthcare/

184. Ingold, John. "A Denver businessman wants to fix America's health care system- by doing your knee replacement in Mexico." *The Colorado Sun*, Feb 3, 2020.

185. Kelly, Kevin. *The Inevitable: Understanding the 12 technological forces that will shape our future*. New York: Penguin Books, 2016. page 60

186. From the Keck School of Medicine of USC. February 20, 2020. https://mphdegree.usc.edu/blog/a-closer-look-at-the-public-health-workforce-crisis/

187. Purtill, Corrine. "Stop Me if you've Heard This One: A Robot and a Team of Irish Scientists Walk into a Senior Living Home." *Time Magazine*, November 4, 2019
https://time.com/longform/senior-care-robot/

188. Davenport, Thomas and Ravi Kalakota. "The potential for artificial intelligence in healthcare." *Future Health J* 6, no. 2(June 2019): 94–98. doi:10.7861/futurehosp.6-2-9

189. Park, Andrea. 7 AI systems outperforming medical experts. *Becker's Hospital Review*, July 1, 2019.
https://www.beckershospitalreview.com/artificial-intelligence/7-ai-systems-outperforming-medical-experts.html

190. "Artificial Intelligence Detects Pediatric Heart Murmurs with Cardiologist-Level Accuracy," presentation at the American Heart Association's Scientific Meeting on Nov 18, 2018

191. Kuo, Weicheng, Christian Häne, Pratik Mukherjee, Jitendra Malik and Esther L. Yuh. "Expert-level detection of acute intracranial hemorrhage on head computed tomography using deep learning." *PNAS* 116, no. 45 (Oct 2019): 22737-22745; October 21, 2019

https://doi.org/10.1073/pnas.1908021116 (Proceedings of the National Academy of Sciences)

192. Milea, Dan, Raymond P. Najjar, Jiang Zhubo, Daniel Ting, Caroline Vasseneix, Xinxing Xu, Masoud Aghsaei Fard et al: Artificial Intelligence to Detect Papilledema from Ocular Fundus photographs. *N Engl J Med* 382, no. 18 (April 2020): 1687-1695. DOI:10.1056/NEJM0a1917130   Epub 2020 Apr 14

193. Niiler, Eric. "An Epidemiologist Sent the First Warning of the Wuhan Virus." *Wired*, Jan 25, 2020. https://www.wired.com/story/ai-epidemiologist-wuhan-public-health-warnings,

194. Perez, Marco V., Kenneth W. Mahaffey, Haley Hedlin, John S. Rumsfeld, Ariadna Garcia, Todd Ferris, Vidhya Balasubramanian et al: "Large-scale Assessment of a Smartwatch to identify Atrial Fibrillation. *N Engl J Med* 381, no. 20 (Nov 2019):1909-1917 doi:10.1056/NEJMoa1901183

195. Obermeyer, Ziad, Brian Powers, Christine Vogeli and Sendhil Mullainathan. "Dissecting racial bias in an algorithm used to manage the health of populations." *Science* 2019: Vol. 366, no. 6464(Oct 2019): 447-453 DOI: 10.1126/science. aax2342

196. Freeman, Karoline, Jacqueline Dinnes, Naomi Chuchu, Yemisi Takwoingi, Sue E Bayliss, Rubeta N. Matin, Abhilash Jain et al: "Algorithm based smart phone apps to assess risk of skin cancer in adults: systematic review of diagnostic accuracy studies." *BMJ* 368, issue.8233 (Feb 2020):m127   doi:10.1136/bmj.m127

197. Morley, Jessica, Luciano Floridi and Ben Goldacre. "The Poor Performance of apps assessing skin cancer." *BMJ* 368, issue. 8233(Feb 2020):m428   doi:10.1136/bmj.m428

198. Miller, Geralyn. "AI and health care are made for each other." *Time Magazine*, Nov 4, 2019
https://time.com/5709346/artificial-intelligence-health/

199. University of Michigan poll on acceptance and attitudes about telemedicine among people age 50-80.
https://ihpi.umich.edu/news/poll-telehealth-visits-have-skyrocketed-older-adults-some-concerns-barriers-remain

200. www.teladochealth.com.

201. Park, Andrea. "75% of Gen Z –and half of baby boomers- make healthcare transactions online." *Becker's Hospital Review,* Feb 24, 2020. https://www.beckershospitalreview.com/consumerism/75-of-gen-z-and-half-of-baby-boom...

202. Dan, Bruce and Roxanne Young. *A Piece of My Mind*. New York: Feeling Fine Programs, 1988. (A series of weekly essays in *JAMA)*

203. Frankel, Allan, Carol Haraden, Frank Federico and Jennifer Lenoci-Edwards. "*A Framework for Safe, Reliable, and Effective Care White Paper."* Cambridge, MA: Institute for Healthcare Improvement and Safe & Reliable Healthcare, 2017) www.ihi.org

204. The Alyssa Hemmelgarn Story.
https://patientsafetymovement.org/advocacy/patients-and-families/patient-advocates/carole-hemmelgarn/ and http://alyssacares.org/alyssas-cause.htm

205. Brooks, Megan. "Pediatrician Suicide Note Reveals Regret Over Fake Vaccination." *Medscape*, Feb 13, 2020. https://www.medscape.com/viewarticle/925249

206. Rappleye, Emily. "Viewpoint: If Vanderbilt nurse is arrested for homicide, leadership should be too." *Becker's Hospital Review*, May 13th, 2019. https://www.beckershospitalreview.com/hospital-management-administration/viewpoint-if-vanderbilt-nurse-is-arrested-for-homicide-leadership-should-be-too.html

207. Reverby, Susan M. (editor). *Tuskegee's Truths: Rethinking the Tuskegee Syphilis Study*. Chapel Hill: University of North Carolina Press; 2000.

208. Masson, Gabrielle. "Cremation of Paul Tyler without family being aware." *Becker's Hospital Review*, February 12, 2020. https://beckershopitalreview.com/post/post-acute-care/nursing-home-patient-dies-is-cre...

209. Helsel, Phil. "New Jersey hospital gives kidney to wrong transplant patient." *NBC News* Nov 27, 2019. https://www.nbcnews.com/news/us-news/new-jersey

210. Orstein, Charles. "Quaids recall twins' drug overdose." *Los Angeles Times*, September 16, 2014. https://www.latimes.com/local/la-me-quaid15jan15-story.html

211. Masson, Gabrielle. "A timeline of all mold-related events at Seattle Children's Hospital." *Becker's Hospital Review*, Feb 28, 2020. https://www.beckershospitalreview.com/infection-control/a-timeline-of-all-mold-related-e...

212. Masson, Gabrielle. "Before mea culpa, Children's Hospital was confident its air systems weren't the source of infection." *The Seattle Times*, November 26, 2019.

213. van Ingen, Jakko, Thomas A. Kohl, Katharina Kranzer, Barbara Hasse, Peter M. Keller, Anna Katarzyna Szafrańska, Doris Hillemann et al: "Global outbreak of severe Mycobacterium chimaera disease after cardiac surgery: a molecular epidemiological study." *The Lancet Infectious Diseases.* Volume 17, Issue 10(Oct 2017):1033-1041 https://doi.org/10.1016/S1473-3099(17)30324-9

214. Moseley, Bruce J., Kimberly O'Malley, Nancy J. Petersen, Terri J. Menke, Baruch A. Brody, David H. Kuykendall, John C. Hollingsworth et al. "A controlled trial of arthroscopic surgery for osteoarthritis of the knee." *N Engl J Med* 347, no.2 (July 2002):81-88. DOI: 10.1056/NEJMoa013259.

215. Niessen, Timothy. "Things we do for no reason." *American College of Physicians,* Annual meeting of the Delaware Chapter. February 8, 2020.

216. Rank, Brian. "Executive Physicals- Bad medicine on three counts." *N Engl J Med* 359, no. 14 (Oct 2008):1424-25. doi:10.1056/NEJMp0806270

217. Ge, Alan and David L Brown. "Assessment of Cardiovascular Diagnostic Tests and Procedures Offered in Executive Screening Programs at Top Ranked Cardiology Hospitals." *JAMA Intern Med* 180, no.4(Jan 2020):586-589 DOI:10.1001/jamainternmed.2019.6607

218. Reilly, Brendan M. "Waste, Worry, and the Seven Sins of Medicine." *N Engl J Med* 382, no.14 (April 2020):1295-1297. doi: 10.1056/NEJMp191703

219. Asher R. "The Seven Sins of Medicine." *Lancet* 2, no. 6574 (Aug 1949):358-60 doi: 10.1016/s0140-6736(49)90090-2

220. Anna Werner. Alabama Couple Struggling after hospital sues over medical debt: "I wish you'd let me die." *CBS News*, February 20th, 2020. https://www.cbsnews.com/news/health-care-costs-alabama-hospital-sues-patient-to-collect-medical-debt-after-appendectomy/

221. Ayla Ellison. *Becker's Hospital Review*, February 3, 2020. https://beckershospitalreview.com/finance/south-carolina-hospital-sued-over-debt-coll

222. Shilts, Randy and William Greider. *And the Band Played On: Politics, People, and the AIDS Epidemic.* New York: Stonewall Inn Editions, 656 pages, Published April 9th, 2000. First published November 1, 1987

223. Wakefield, Andrew J., Simon H. Murch, Andrew Anthony, J. Linell, D.M. Casson, M. Malik, M. Berelowitz M., et al. "Ileal-lymphoid-nodular hyperplasia, nonspecific colitis, and pervasive developmental disorder in children." *Lancet* 351, issue 9 (Feb 1998) 637-41. (Paper retracted by Lancet in February 2010) https://doi.org/10.1016/S0140-6736(97)11096-0

224. Rao, Sathyanrayana T.S. and Andrade Chittaranjan. "The MMR Vaccine and autism: Sensation, refutation, retracted fraud." *Indian J Psychiatry* 53, no. 2(Apr-June 2011):95-96. http://www.indianjpsychiatry.org/text.asp?2011/53/2/95/82529

225. Fiore, Kristine. 'Dead Doctors Don't Lie'-Pediatrician threatened." *MedPage Today*, January 21, 2020. https://www.medpagetoday.com/special-reports/exclusives/84446

226. Vaidya, Anuja. "Hospital worker fired for refusing flu shot not victim of religious bias, court rules." *Becker's Health Reviews*, February 18, 2020. https://www.beckershealthreviews.com/legal-regulatory-issues/hospital-worker-fired-for-r...

227. Eban, Katherine. *Bottle of Lies: The Inside Story of the Generic Drug Boom.* New York: Harper Collins, 2019

228. Gibson, Rosemary and Janardan Prasad Singh. *China Rx: Exposing the Risks of America's Dependence on China for Medicine.* Prometheus Books, April 17, 2018, 304 pages

229. Hsu, Heather E., Rui Wang, Carly Broadwell, Kelly Horan, Robert Jin, Chanu Rhee and Grace M. Lee. "Association Between Federal Value-Based incentive Programs and Health Care-Associated Infection Rates in Safety-Net and Non-Safety Net Hospitals." *JAMA Netw Open* 3, no.7(July 2020): e209700 doi:10.1001/jamanetworkopen.2020.9700

230. History - Edward Jenner – *BBC.* www.bbc.co.uk›history›historic_figures›jenner_ed...

231. Close, William T. *Ebola: A Documentary Novel of its First Explosion.* New York: Ballantine Books, 1995.

232. Hargreaves, Allison L., Glen Nowak, Paula M. Frew, Alan R. Hinman, Walter A. Orenstein, Judith Mendel, Ann Aikin et al. "Pediatrics Adherence to Timely Vaccinations in the United States."

Pediatrics 145, no.3 (March 2020): e20190783
https://doi.org/10.1542/peds.2019-0783

233. Pronovost, Peter, Dale Needham, Sean Berenholtz, David Sinopoli, Haitau Chu, Sara Cosgrove, Bryan Sexton et al "An Intervention to Decrease Catheter-Related Bloodstream Infections in the ICU." *N Engl J Med* 355 (2006):2725-2732 DOI: 10.1056/NEJMoa061115

234. Preventing C. diff infections through training, technology and innovation. Link to C. difficile Colitis video on *YouTube;* (produced by Christiana Care on Sep 24, 2013).
https://www.google.com/url?sa=t&rct=j&q=&esrc=s&source=web&cd=2&cad=rja&uact=8&ved=2ahUKEwiQ2Ob7yL3nAhUQyFkKHVe9BHkQwqsBMAF6BAgKEAQ&url=https%3A%2F%2Fwww.youtube.com%2Fwatch%3Fv%3DR2zSwkBP2GA&usg=AOvVaw08ihe1hGFU0Dsy40zBjcZ-

235. Stout, Janet E., Robert R. Muder, Sue Mietzner, Marilyn M. Wagener, Mary Beth Perri, Kathleen DeRoos, Donna Goodrich et al. "Role of environmental surveillance in determining the risk of hospital-acquired legionellosis: a national surveillance study with clinical correlations." *Infect Control Hosp Epidemiol* 28, no. 7(July 2007)818-24 DOI: 10.1086/518754 Epub 2007 Jun 5, 2007

236. Panwalker, Anand P. and Elizabeth Fuhse. "Nosocomial Mycobacterium gordonae Pseudo-infection from Contaminated Ice Machines." *Infection Control and Hospital Epidemiology* 7, no.2 (Feb 1986):67-70. DOI:10.1017/s0195

237. William H. Whyte "Is Anybody Listening?" *Fortune Magazine*, September 1950.

238. Kapoor, Alok, Terry Field, Steven Handler, Kimberly Fisher, Cassandra Saphirak, Sybil Crawford, Hassan Fouayzi et al. "Adverse events in Long-Term Care Residents transitioning From Hospital Back to Nursing Home." *JAMA Intern Med* 179, no.9(July 2019): 1254-1261. doi:10.1001/jamainternmed.2019.2005

239. "List of Confused Drug Names." *Institute for Safe Medication Practices*, February 28, 2019.
https://www.ismp.org/recommendations/confused-drug-names-list

240. Bergen, Gwen, Mark R. Stevens and Elizabeth R. Burns. Falls and injuries among adults aged >65 years- United States, 2014. *Morb Mortal Wkly Rep. (MMWR)* 65, no. 37(Sept 2016): 993-998. doi:10.15585/mmwr.mm6537a2

241. Hartholt, Klaas A., Robin Lee, Elizabeth Burns and Ed F. van Beeck. "Mortality from falls among US adults Aged 75 years or Older, 2000-2016." *JAMA* 321, no. 21(June 2019):2131-2133 doi:10.1001/jama.2019.4185

242. Greeley, Adela M., Elizabeth P. Tanner, Selene Mak, Meron M. Begashaw, Isomi M. Miake-Lye and Paul G. Shekelle. "Sitters as a Patient Safety Strategy to Reduce Hospital Falls." *Ann Intern Med* 172, no.5, (Mar 2020): 317-324 doi:10.7326/M19-2628

243. Luo, Jing, Martin Kulldorff, Ameet Sarpatwari, Ajinkya Pawar and Aaron S. Kesselheim. "Variation in Prescription Drug prices by Retail Pharmacy Type; A National Cross-sectional study." *Ann Intern Med* 171, no. 9 (Nov 2019): 605-611. DOI:10.7326/M18-1138

244. Gooch, Kelly. Quoting Andre Machado from the Cleveland Clinic's Neurologic Institute. *Becker's Hospital Review*, Dec 19, 2019.

https://www.beckershospitalreview.com/quality/8-clinical-leaders-share-tips-for-improving-the-patient-experience.html

245.   Silverman, Mark E., T. Jock Murray and Charles S. Bryan. *The Quotable Osler (revised edition)* 2008. The American College of Physicians, Versa Press. (Live in the present p 37)

246.   Ibid. (The practice of medicine is what you make it. P 51)

247.   Ibid. (The clinician who keeps an eye on the watch while in the wards, is rarely successful. p 54)

248.   Ibid. (Listen to the patient. P 98)

249.   Ibid. (On having a hobby. P 189)

250.   Ibid. (Lifelong learning. P 206)

251.   Dr. Gary Marshall (University of Louisville) speaking at the *Communicable Disease Summit* in Newark, Delaware, on December 9, 2019.

252.   "If I cannot do great things, I can do small things in a great way." Martin Luther King Jr.

253.   Landro, Laura. "Building Team Spirit: Nurses hesitate to challenge doctors even when doctors are ordering the wrong drug or operating on the wrong limb. Interview with Peter Pronovost, author of book on safety." *The Wall Street Journal*, Feb 16, 2010.
https://www.wsj.com/articles/SB10001424052748704431404575067921122148064

254. Pronovost, Peter and Eric Vohr. *Safe Patients, Safe Hospitals: How One Doctor's Checklist Can help US Change Health Care from Inside Out.* New York: Hudson Street Press, 2010. 282 pages

255. Storytellerdoc. "This is a real problem in our ER. This is a real problem nationwide." *KevinMD,* Jan 21, 2020.
https://www.kevinmd.com/blog/2020/01/this-is-a-real-pro

256. Pothen, Meril. "Health Policy Poets Light Up Twitter for Valentine's Day" - *Medscape* - Feb 18, 2020.
https://www.medscape.com/viewarticle/925372

257. Spellberg, *Brad. Broken, Bankrupt and Dying: How to Solve the Great American Healthcare Rip-off.* Carson City, Nevada: Lioncrest Publishing, 2020.

258. Hrynowski, Zach. "Several Issues Tie as Most Important in 2020 Election." *Gallup Poll.* January 13, 2020
https://news.gallup.com/poll/276932/several-issues-tie-important-2020-election.aspx

259. Alter, Charlotte. *The Ones we've been waiting for: How a new generation of leaders will transform America.* Viking, Penguin Random House, Feb 18, 2020.

260. Larson, Chris. "Disruptive Innovation Theory: What It Is & 4 Key Concepts." *Harvard Business Review,* November 15, 2016.
https://online.hbs.edu/blog/post/4-keys-to...

261. Gawande, Atul. The Hot Spotters. *New Yorker,* January 24, 2011 https://www.newyorker.com/magazine/2011/01/24/the-hot-spotters

262. Blum, Michael R., Henning Øien, Harris L. Carmichael, Paul Heidenreich, Douglas K. Owens and Jeremy D. Goldhaber-Fiebert. "Cost-Effectiveness of Transitional Care Services After Hospitalization with Heart Failure. *Ann Intern Med* 172, no.4 (Feb 2020):248-257. Doi:10.7326/M19-1980

263. Finkelstein, Amy, Annetta Zhou, Sarah Taubman and Joseph Doyle. "Health Care hot spotting- A randomized, controlled trial." *N Engl J Med* 382 (Jan 2020):152-162
https://www.nejm.org/doi/full/10.1056/NEJMsa1906848

264. Maddux, Duggan. "Entering the voice era: From Scribes to Scribble." *Acumen Physician Solutions*, July 16, 2018.
https://acumenmd.com/blog/entering-the-voice-era-from-scribes-to-scribble/

265. Bechtel, Christine. "As a patient, I never understood the heartbreakingly human toll our system takes on clinicians." *KevinMD*, August 13, 2019. https://www.kevinmd.com/blog/2019/08/as-a-patient-i-never-understood-the-heartbreaking...

266. James, Brent C. and Lucy A Savitz. "How Intermountain trimmed health care costs through robust quality improvement Efforts." *Health Affairs* 30 no. 6 (June 2011):1185-91
https://doi.org/10.1377/hlthaff.2011.0358

267. Greenleaf, R.K. *The Servant as Leader*. Indianapolis, IN: The Robert K. Greenleaf Center. 1991. Originally published in 1970, by Robert K. Greenleaf.

268. Peter Ubel. "What Socialized Medicine Would Mean for Your Health." *Forbes*, Nov 21, 2018
https://www.forbes.com/sites/peterubel/2018/11/21/...

269. Jha, Ashish, Jonathan B. Perlin, Kenneth W. Kizer and R. Adams Dudley. "Effect of the transformation of the Veterans Affairs Health Care System on the quality of care." *New Engl J Med* 348, no. 22 (2003) p18-27.

270. O'Hanlon, Claire, Christina Huang, Elizabeth Sloss, Rebecca Anhang Price, Peter Hussey, Carrie Farmer and Courtney Gidengil. "Comparing VA and Non-VA Quality of Care: A Systematic Review." *J Gen Intern Med*, 32, no. 1, (January 2017) p 105–121. doi: 10.1007/s11606-016-3775-2.

271. Trivedi, Amal N, Sierra Matula, Isomi Miake-Lye, Peter A. Glassman, Paul Shekelle, Steven Asch. "Systematic review: comparison of the quality of medical care in Veterans Affairs and non-Veterans Affairs settings." *Med Care* 49, no. 1 (January 2011) p76-88 doi: 10.1097/MLR.0b013e3181f53575.

272. Anhang, Rebecca Price, Elizabeth M. Sloss, Mathew Cefalu, Carrie M. Farmer and Peter S. Hussey. "Comparing Quality of Care in Veterans Affairs and Non-Veterans Affairs Settings." *J Gen Intern Med* 33, no.10 (Oct 2018) 1631-1638. Doi: 10.1007/s11606-018-4433-7.

273. Panwalker, Anand. *The Place of Cold Water: A Memoir*. Newark, Delaware: CreateSpace, 2017.

274. Pinsky, William. "The importance of International Medical graduates in the United States." *Annals Intern Med* Vol 166, no. 11, (June 6, 2017)

275. Jenkins, Tania M. *Doctor's Orders: The Making of Status Hierarchies in an Elite Program*. New York: Columbia University Press, 2019.

276. Verghese, Abraham. *My Own Country: A Doctor's Story of a town and its people in the Age of AIDS*. New York: Simon and Schuster, 1994.

277. Verghese, Abraham. *Cutting for Stone*. New York: Alfred A. Knoff, 2009.

278. Haefner, Morgan. "Nursing home chain settles false billing allegations for $9.5M." *Becker's Hospital Review*, March 2, 2020
https://www.beckershospitalreview.com/legal-regulatory-issues/nursing-home-chain-settles-...

279. D'Ambrosio, Amanda. "Scripts for Dead Patients…" *MedPage Today*, Jan 24, 2020.
https://www.medpagetoday.com/publichealthpolicy/ethics/84515?xid=nl_badpractice_202

280. Haefner, Morgan. "Tennessee physician settles allegations of inflating NP charges." *Becker's Hospital Review*, January 28th, 2020.
https://www.beckershospitalreview.com/legal-regulatory-issues/tennessee-physician-settle...

281. Drees, Jackie. "Owners of telemedicine companies charged in $56M Medicare fraud scheme." *Becker's Hospital Review*, February 6th, 2020.
https://www.beckershospitalreview.com/legal-regulatory-issues/owners-of-telemedicine-co...

282. Ellison, Ayla. California physician sentenced to prison over $700K in fraudulent billings. *Becker's Hospital Review*, Feb 25th, 2020.
https://www.beckershospitalreview.com/legal-regulatory-issues/california-physician-sentenced-to-prison-over-700k-in-fraudulent-billings.html

283. "Texas Doctor Found Guilty for Role in $325 Million Health Care Fraud Scheme Involving False Diagnoses of Life-Long Diseases." *The US Department of Justice.* January 15, 2020. https://www.justice.gov/opa/pr/texas-doctor-found-guilty-role-325-million-health-care-fraud-scheme-involving-false-diagnoses

284. Ellison, Ayla. "Mississippi hospital owner defrauded Medicare of $10.8M, jury finds." *Becker's Hospital Review,* March 17, 2020. https://www.beckershospitalreview.com/legal-regulatory-issues/mississippi-hospital-owner...

285. Ellison, Ayla. "Florida physician charged in $681M billing fraud scheme." *Becker's Hospital Review,* August 3rd, 2020. https://www.beckershospitalreview.com/legal-regulatory-issues/florida-physician-charged-in-681m-billing-fraud-scheme.html

286. Diaz, Johnny. "Florida Doctor Bilked $26 Million From Health Insurers, Officials Say." *New York Times,* February 15, 2020.

287. Ellison, Ayla. "New York physician sentenced to prison for role in $30M billing scheme." *Becker's Hospital Review,* Dec 12, 2019. https://www.beckershospitalreview.com/legal-regulatory-issues/new-york-physician-sentenced-to-prison-for-role-in-30m-billing-scheme-121219.html

288. Held, Colleen. "UNMH was told about inferior treatments, witnesses say." *Albuquerque Journal,* December 15, 2019. https://www.abqjournal.com/1401588/unmh-was-told-about-inferior-treatments-witnesses-say.html

289. Garrity, McKenzie. "Patients allege overcharge for copies of their records." *Becker's Hospital Review,* February 18, 2020

https://www.beckershospitalreview.com/ehrs/patients-say-medical-records-company-overc

290. Vigdor, Neil. "It Paid Doctors Kickbacks. Now, Novartis Will Pay a $678 Million Settlement." *NY Times,* July 1, 2020.
https://www.nytimes.com/2020/07/01/business/...

291. Miller, Jessica. "Former Utah nurse pleads guilty to stealing painkillers and infecting seven patients with hepatitis C." *The Salt Lake Tribune,* September 26, 2019.
https://www.sltrib.com/news/2019/09/25/former-utah-nurse-pleads

ACKNOWLEDGMENTS

My late wife, Asha, inspired me to write this book. Numerous reviewers spent hours reading the manuscript, checking every punctuation mark and hyphen and calling me out when my statements could not be corroborated. Some did that during their vacations or time meant for family. Their polite challenges and corrections were invaluable as I waded through rather complex territory. I am deeply indebted to Vijay Abhyankar, Vijaya Balchandani, David Bercaw, Bala Carver, Avinash Chitnis, Joan Delfattore, Shefali Kapoor Dhir, Kumar Fanse, Christopher Haines, Carole Hemmelgarn, Sitara Jabeen, Pradip Khaladkar, Omar Khan, Bennett Lorber, James Malow, Richard Plotzker, Vijay Sathe, Chuck Selvaggio, Brad Spellberg, Wesley White and Dean Winslow.

Content experts David Donohue, Jennifer Goldstein, Terry Horton, Mausumee Hussain, Vishal Patel, Reinhard Roos, Scott Siegel and Lauren Tavani reviewed portions of the book and provided valuable insights. I am so grateful for their corrections and guidance.

I am grateful to Lois Hoffman, a consummate professional, who helped me launch my first book *The Place of Cold Water* in 2017, guided me through this effort as well and my son, Sandeep, who took care of the technical glitches whenever I needed his expertise.

www.ingramcontent.com/pod-product-compliance
Lightning Source LLC
Chambersburg PA
CBHW060824220526
45466CB00003B/965